THE 7-DAY
FERTILITY MEAL PLAN
FOR WOMEN
OVER 40

Nutrition and Diet Book to Balance Hormones, Improve Egg Quality, Reduce Inflammation, and Quicken Pregnancy

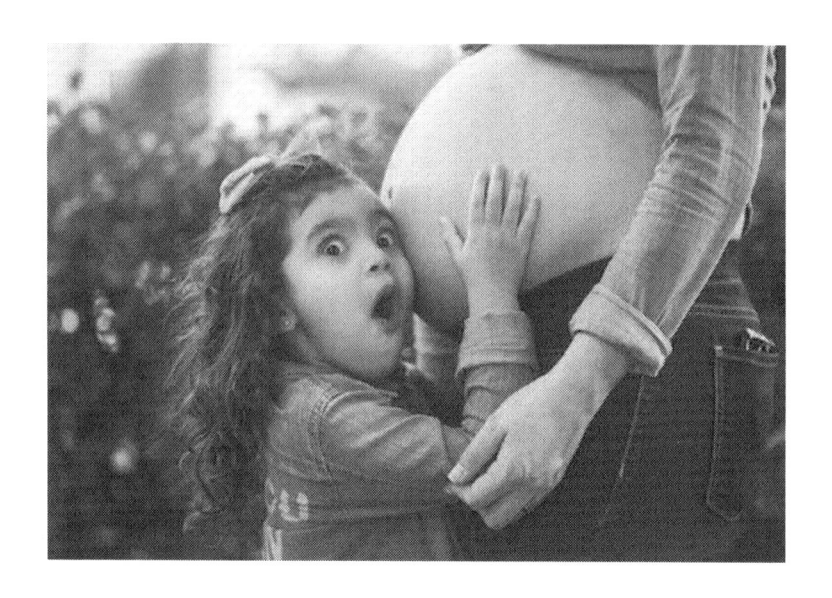

DR. KADEN WINTON

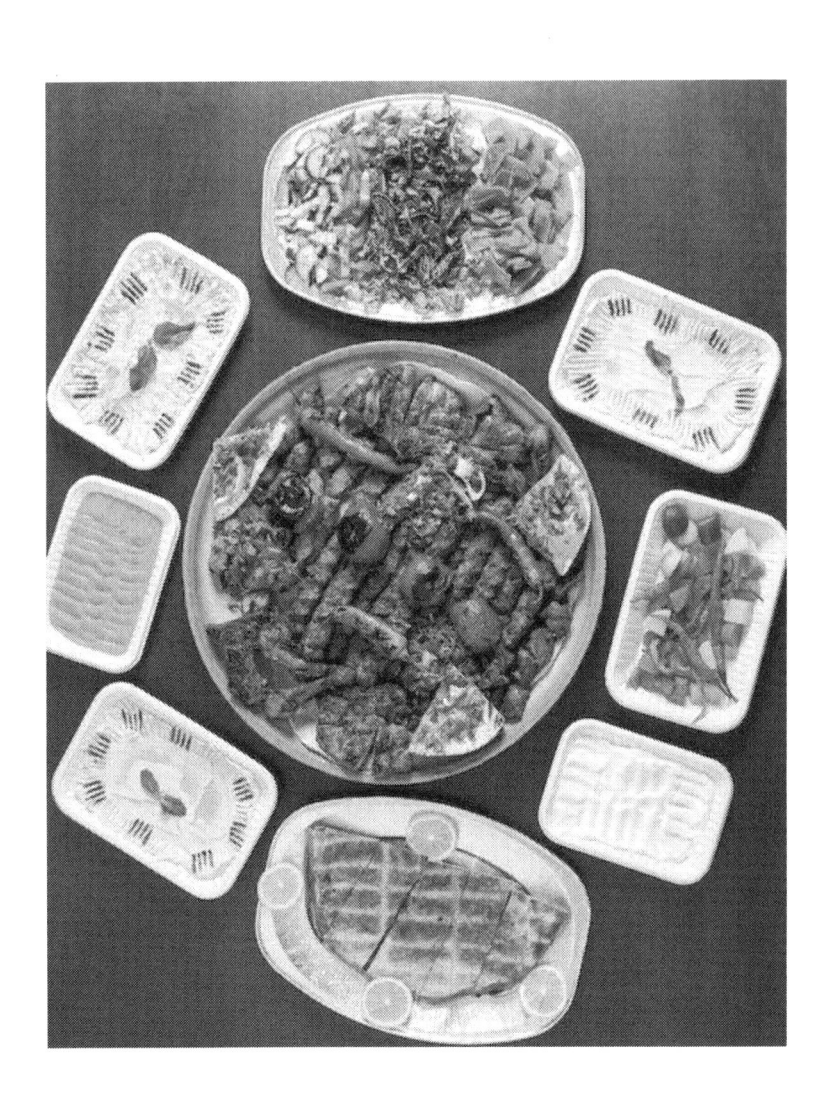

Copyright © 2023 KADEN WINTON

All rights reserved. No part of this publication may be reproduced, stored in a retrieval system, or transmitted in any form or by any means, electronic, mechanical, photocopying, recording, or otherwise, without the publisher's prior written permission.

This book is sold subject to the condition that it shall not, by way of trade or otherwise, be lent, re-sold, hired out, or otherwise circulated without the publisher's prior consent in any form of binding or cover other than that in which it is published and without a similar condition, including this condition, being imposed on the subsequent purchaser.

The views expressed in this book are those of the author and do not necessarily reflect the views of the publisher.

Table of Contents

Introduction 11
Chapter One 17
   Menopause Diet and Hormones 17
   How significant is your diet? 18
   The objectives and advantages of a fertility meal plan 21
   Key Nutrients for a Quicker and healthy pregnancy 24
Chapter Two 29
   Fertility Meal Plan Guidelines 29
CHAPTER THREE 33
   The Fertility Diet Cookbook; Recipes Meal Plan and Meal Preparation 33
   Day 1 34
   Breakfast: 34
   Ingredients 34
   Preparation 35
   Meal Preparation Tips 36
   Note 37
   Lunch 38
   Ingredients 38
   Preparation 39
   Meal Preparation Tips 41
   Note 41
   Dinner 42
   Ingredients: 42
   Preparation 43

Meal Preparation Tips:	44
Note	45
Snack	46
Ingredients	46
Procedure	47
Preparation Tips	48
Note	49
Day 2	49
Breakfast	49
Ingredients	50
Preparation	50
Meal Preparation Tips	51
Note	52
Lunch	53
Ingredients	53
Procedure	54
Meal Preparation Tips	55
Note	56
Dinner	56
Ingredients	57
Procedure:	58
Meal Preparation Tips	59
Note	60
Snacks	61
Ingredients	61
Preparation	62
Meal Preparation Tips	63

Note 64
Day 3 64
Breakfast 64
Ingredients 65
Procedure 65
Meal Preparation Tips 66
Note 67
Lunch 68
Ingredients 68
Procedure 69
Meal Preparation Tips 71
Note 71
Dinner 72
Ingredients 72
Procedure 73
Meal Preparation Tips 75
Note: 76
Snack 76
Ingredients 77
Preparation 77
Preparation Tips: 78
Note 79
Day 4 80
Breakfast 80
Ingredients 80
Preparation 81
Meal Preparation Tips 81

Note	82
Lunch	83
Ingredients	83
Procedure	84
Meal Preparation Tips	85
Note	86
Dinner	87
Ingredients	87
Procedure	88
Meal Preparation Tips	89
Note	90
Snack	91
Procedure	92
Meal Preparation Tips	93
Note	93
Day 5	94
Ingredients	94
Procedure	95
Meal Preparation Tips	96
Note	97
Lunch	98
Ingredients:	98
Procedure	99
Meal Preparation Tips	100
Note	101
Dinner	102
Ingredients	103

Procedure 104
Meal Preparation Tips 105
Snack 106
Ingredients 107
Procedure 107
Preparation Tips: 108
Note 109
Day 6 110
Breakfast 110
Ingredients 111
Procedure 111
Meal Preparation Tips: 112
Note 113
Lunch 114
Ingredients 114
Procedure 115
Preparation Tips 117
Note 118
Dinner 118
Ingredients 119
Preparation 120
Preparation tips 121
Note 122
Snack 123
Ingredients 123
Procedure 123
Meal Preparation Tips 125

Note 125
Day 7 126
Breakfast: Banana Pancakes with Maple Syrup and Walnuts 126
Ingredients 126
Procedure 127
Meal Preparation Tips: 128
Note 129
Lunch 130
Ingredients 130
Procedure 131
Meal Preparation Tips: 132
Note 133
Dinner 133
Ingredients 134
Procedure 135
Meal Preparation Tips 137
Note 137
Snack 138
Ingredients 138
Procedure 139
Meal Preparation Tips: 140
Note 140
Extra Methods to Enhance Fertility 141
CONCLUSION 144

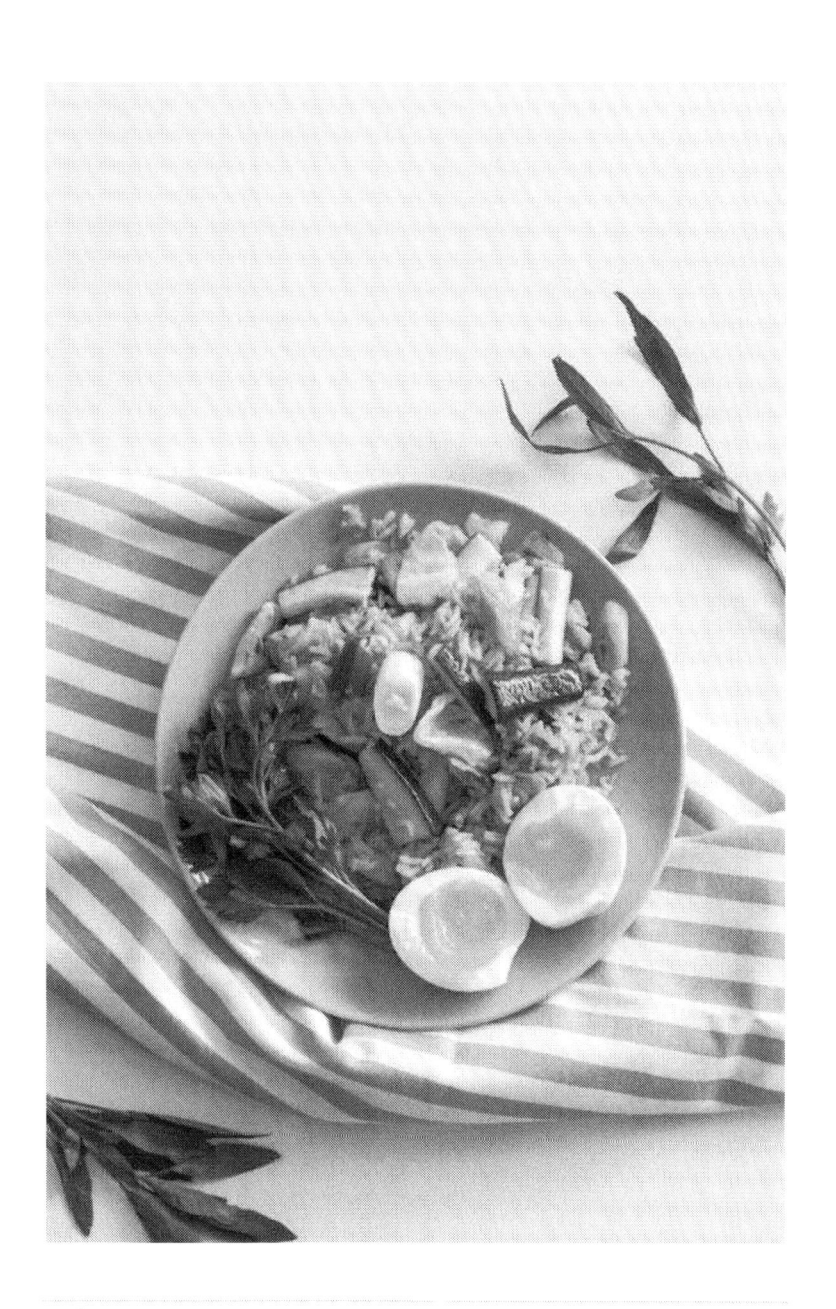

Introduction

Emma was a banker who lived in a small village with her husband. She had always aspired to become a mother, but her hopes began to wane as time passed. Emma's soul began to disintegrate after being informed she was infertile and facing countless disappointments, Emma's spirit started to crumble. However, little did she know that her life was about to change in the most unexpected way.

Emma got lost in the depths of her despair; she spent the majority of her nights wondering if she was plagued by infertility.

On a beautiful Wednesday evening, she came across a social media post I had made. She clicked, read my article, and then purchased my book, "The 7-Day Fertility Meal Plan for Women over 40." The book guaranteed another way to deal with fertility, mixing nourishment and comprehensive way of life decisions. Emma decided to give it a shot out of curiosity. She thought it was worth going after if there was even hope.

With a renewed sense of determination, Emma set out on her journey. She carefully followed each meal plan page, enjoying the delicious recipes and nourishing ingredients. From the energetic greens of her morning smoothies to the healthy grains and lean proteins that graced her plate, each nibble turned into an image of restored trust.

Weeks transformed into months, and Emma found an inconspicuous shift inside herself. She started to feel a recently discovered imperativeness flowing through her veins. Her well-being improved as a whole, and her energy levels skyrocketed. Maybe the painstakingly created meal plan had stirred lethargic powers inside her body.

However, the real miracle occurred within Emma's womb. She discovered the unimaginable after years of heartbreak and dashed hopes: she was pregnant. She realized that the 7-day fertility meal plan had provided her with her long-awaited miracle, and she was overcome with joy and gratitude.

Emma's pregnancy progressed without a hitch, and she treasured every moment. Her precious new life was now being nurtured by the same nutrients that had nourished her body. Knowing that she had discovered a potent secret that had the potential to alter the lives of numerous other women just like her, she embraced each day with gratitude.

The transformation of Emma was widely reported. Ladies from varying backgrounds, tested with fertility battles, contacted her, looking for direction and trust. Emma became a reference point of light, sharing her story and the groundbreaking insight in "The 7-Day Fertility Meal Plan for Women over 40."

Emma's baby girl was brought into the world as time elapsed, filling her existence with indefinable love. A personal triumph, Emma's transformation from barren to blossoming is a testament to the power of nourishment for the mind and body.

Emma recommended her book which have transformed her fertility struggles to her friends months later, the same book which helped her unlock her womb, improved her eating habits and cooking skills, and in no time numerous people discovered their resilience and hoped through her words and experiences.

The story of Emma became a constant reminder that miracles are possible and that even the most difficult times can result in the best outcomes.

As a result, women of today continue to be inspired by the story of Emma's journey. Remember that the most unexpected places can sometimes hold the key to fulfilling our deepest desires. "The 7-Day Fertility Meal Plan for Women Over 40" holds the key to turning barrenness into blossoming life and dreams into reality.

As ladies enter their forties, another part of life starts — one loaded up with shrewdness, development, and the acknowledgment that caring for oneself is fundamental. Among the mainstays of taking care of oneself, nutrition is a valuable asset that can shape the direction of a lady's prosperity. In this book, we discuss the compelling significance of nutrition for women over 40 and demonstrate how nourishing the body can lead to a world of vitality, resilience, and vibrant health.

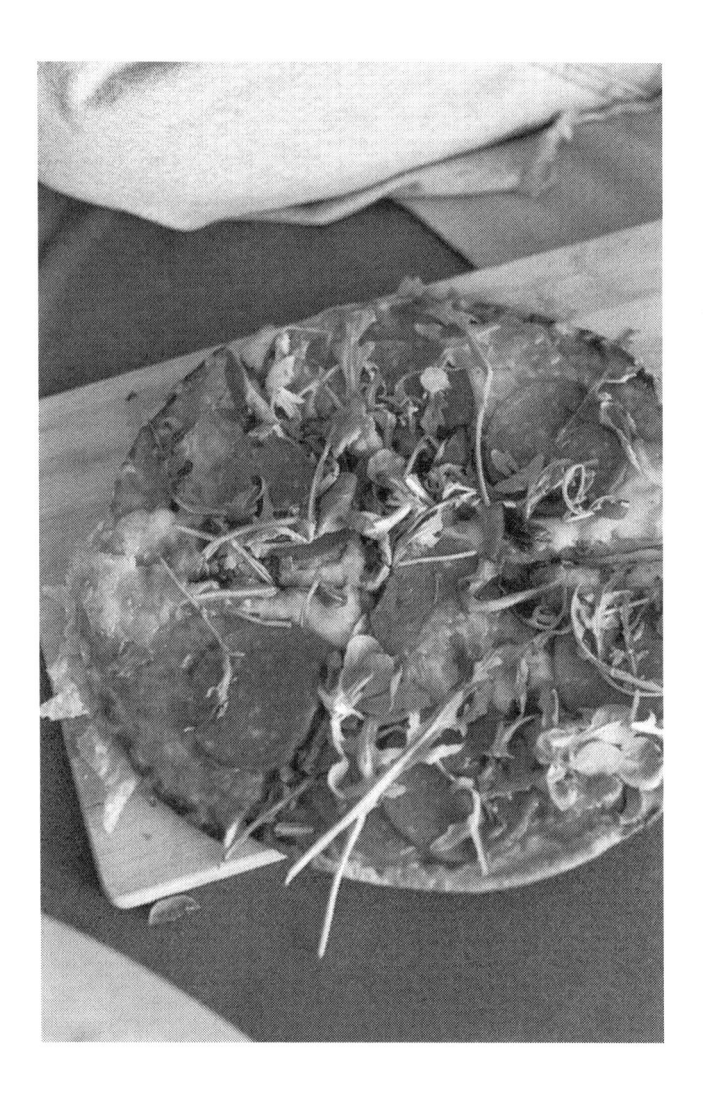

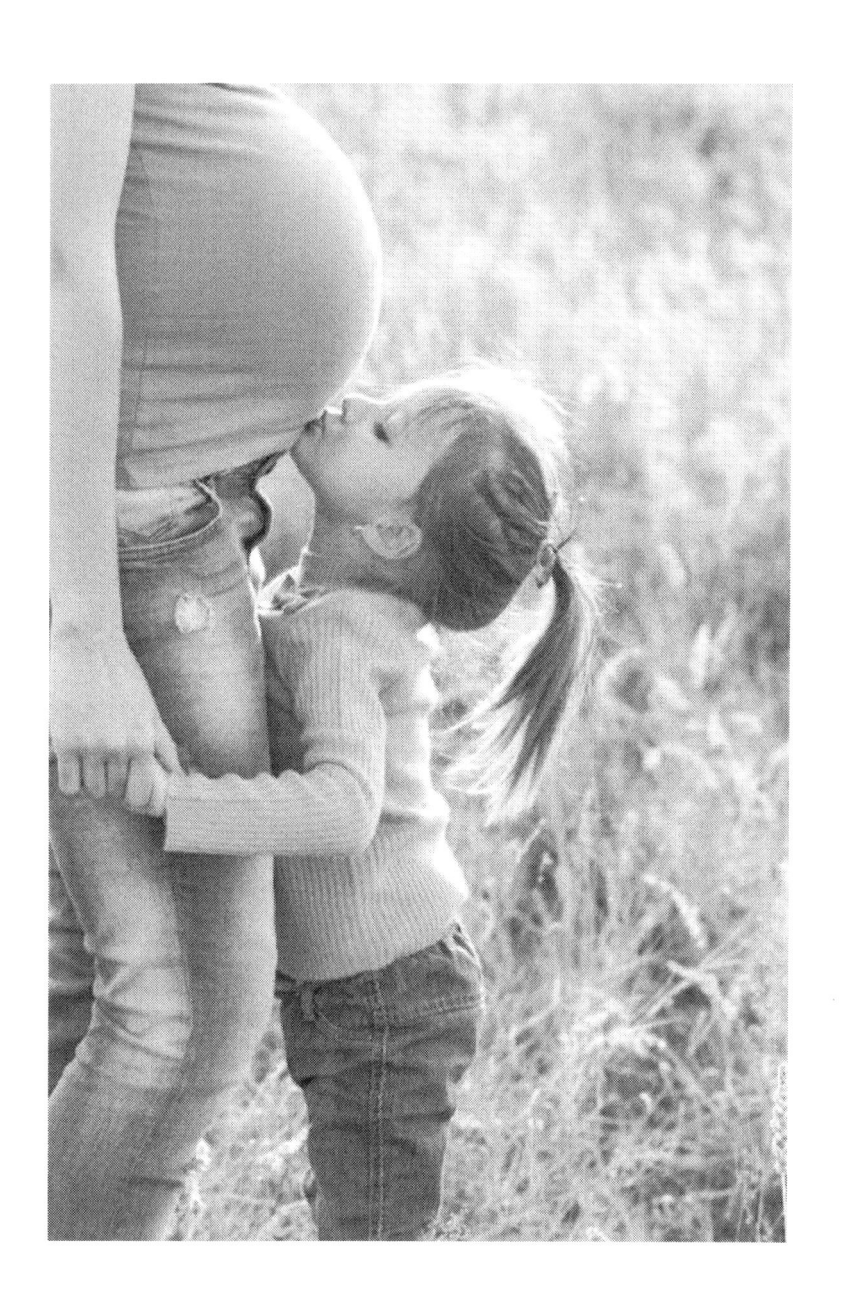

Chapter One

Menopause Diet and Hormones

Transitioning into menopause is one of the most important aspects of a woman's life after age 40. When it comes to controlling hormonal fluctuations and reducing the symptoms that come with them, nutrition plays a crucial role. Flaxseed, soy, and legume phytoestrogens can help regulate hormone levels and alleviate hot flashes, mood swings, and sleep disturbances. Ideal nutrition during this stage engages ladies to explore this extraordinary period with effortlessness and imperativeness.

As ladies nimbly enter their forties and then some, focusing on nourishment becomes a fundamental mainstay of caring for oneself. Women can embrace the process of aging with vitality, resiliency, and unwavering health by eating well. A well-rounded and nutrient-rich diet has significant advantages for women over 40, including hormone balance, bone strength, heart health, and cognitive function. By bridging the force of nourishment, ladies can open their maximum capacity, transmitting splendor at each phase of life. Remember that each bite is a chance to nourish, reenergize, and thrive—so embrace it and your brilliance.

How significant is your diet?

If you're trying to conceive, you might wonder if there is a fertility diet you should follow to have a better chance of getting pregnant quickly. The term "diet" has come to be associated with both good and bad foods due to the prevalence of weight loss programs, and we appear to be losing our sense of reality regarding the foods we consume.

Many couples actively trying to conceive are probably very busy working couples who rarely have time to cook or think about what they eat. Fast foods frequently contain a lot of salt, fat, chemicals, and sugar.

Fertility is an entire body event, and just glancing at your eating regimen in seclusion from any remaining perspectives would be extremely off-base, and this ought to be checked out related to different parts of your way of life. However, the foods you consume can affect your chances of getting pregnant.

There are various straightforward standards of an eating regimen for fertility, and these are pointed toward rebalancing the couples' dietary patterns while including food varieties which, when joined with different strategies, will assist with further developing fertility.

Right off the bat, a detox may be valuable to guarantee that you give your stomach-related framework a rest. The body is frequently dealing with toxins that may have come from smoking, drinking, a poor diet, or even the environment. This is prudent for everyone, as sperm creation improves when the eating routine is tidied up.

Next, try to include seasonal, organically-grown foods whenever possible. But don't worry about this. Ensure that your fruits and vegetables have been thoroughly washed or peeled if you cannot afford organic. Avoid eating foods with artificial additives and eat foods which are as close to their natural state as possible. (ie not processed) This means choosing butter over margarine and sugar (if necessary) over artificial sweeteners.

Old Chinese medication has a few highly healthy standards regarding an eating regimen for fertility and what can have an emotional meaning for the body's organs. It exhorts adjusting the soluble and acidic food sources which we eat as an unevenness one way or the other can be adverse.

Supplements are not a substitute for a healthy diet; some couples believe taking supplements will make them less concerned about eating. Making up for a terrible eating routine isn't equivalent to improving a decent one. Our bodies cannot function properly if we eat poorly, and food that is bad for us often makes toxins, so the body spends more energy trying to deal with the consequences than trying to conceive.

Luckily, the body answers rapidly once an eating regimen for fertility is presented, and you ought to roll out sure improvements towards eating healthy. You should notice a general improvement in your health and vitality as the body becomes receptive for conception.

The objectives and advantages of a fertility meal plan

Becoming a mother is a remarkable and deeply personal one for women. Along this way, a fertility meal plan arises as a vital partner, offering ladies an unmistakable means to help their reproductive well-being, upgrade fertility, and sustain their bodies. We discuss the transformative advantages of a fertility meal plan in this book, giving women the confidence and strength to embrace their fertility and embark on motherhood.

1. Creating a Balance of Hormones:

A fertility meal plan aims to help women achieve hormonal equilibrium. The meal plan provides the essential building blocks for hormonal equilibrium by incorporating foods high in nutrient density and antioxidants, vitamins, and minerals. Adjusting chemicals upholds regular periods, ideal ovulation, and the general working of the Reproductive framework, improving the probability of effective origination.

2. Providing Essential Dietary Needs:

A fertility meal plan aims to provide the body with essential nutrients that help with reproduction. Key supplements like folate, iron, calcium, and omega-3 unsaturated fats are critical in supporting fertility. Folate helps with Healthy fetal development, iron supports proper oxygenation and fertility, calcium reinforces the uterine coating, and omega-3 unsaturated fats improve conceptive capability. Women can help their bodies thrive in the pursuit of motherhood by consuming foods high in these nutrients.

3. Promoting Body Confidence and Weight Management:

Keeping a healthy weight is essential to fertility, and a fertility meal plan offers help in accomplishing and keeping up with the ideal weight. The meal plan helps women reach their weight management goals by emphasizing balanced nutrition, portion control, and mindful eating. Maintaining a healthy weight improves hormonal balance and boosts self-esteem and confidence in one's body, fostering a favorable environment for conception and supporting the motherhood journey.

4. **Promoting Emotional Health and Reducing Stress:**
The infertility journey can be emotionally taxing, frequently accompanied by anxiety and stress. A well-designed fertility meal plan addresses this by including foods that improve emotional well-being and reduce stress. Meals high in nutrients help maintain a stable mood, give you more energy, and make you feel full and satisfied. The meal plan provides women with the resilience and strength to navigate the emotional aspects of the fertility journey by nourishing the mind and body.

5. **Self-care and empowerment are embraced:**

As women embark on their fertility journey, a fertility meal plan encourages them to practice self-care and empower themselves. Ladies function in their conceptive well-being by focusing on nourishment and making careful decisions about their consumption. Women can take control of their bodies and make choices that help them achieve their fertility goals thanks to the meal plan, which transforms into a tool for self-empowerment.

A fertility meal plan fills in as a directing light for ladies, enabling them to embrace their fertility and embark on the excursion towards parenthood with certainty and essentialness. The meal plan becomes a transformative partner on the path to motherhood by maintaining hormonal equilibrium, providing the body with essential nutrients, supporting weight management, fostering emotional well-being, and encouraging self-care. As ladies embrace their fertility, they saddle the strength inside, becoming guards of life's most significant miracle— demonstrating the fantastic power in their grasp and hearts.

Key Nutrients for a Quicker and healthy pregnancy

As women get older, their fertility naturally declines. This makes it much more critical to eat well to keep up with great conceptive thriving. Even though eating a balanced diet is essential, some basic nutrients can help pregnant women over 40 get pregnant. As you continue reading, we review these fundamental nutrients and their specific benefits for fertility growth.

1. Folate

Ladies of any age need the mineral folate, otherwise called nutrient B9; however, pregnant ladies particularly need it. Folate reduces congenital disabilities and helps normalize fetal development. Ladies beyond 40 years old who are pregnant should consume adequate folate to guarantee the child's ideal formation. Consuming foods high in folate, such as vegetables, citrus fruits, propped grains, and blended greens, is recommended. Since folic acid absorption decreases with age, supplements may also be recommended.

2. Iron

Iron is expected all through the body, including the Reproductive system, to create oxygen and healthy red platelets. You need to consume sufficient iron for regular periods and avoid iron deficiency, which can hurt fertility. Iron can be tracked down in braised oats, spinach, lean red meat, poultry, fish, beans, lentils, braised oats, and lentils. Iron ingestion can be improved by joining iron-rich food sources with L-ascorbic acid sources.

3. Calcium

Calcium is fundamental for Healthy bones and, generally speaking, prosperity. Calcium affects fertility by supporting standard uterine capability, regulating chemical levels, and working with treatment. Calcium can prevent endometriosis and polycystic ovary syndrome (PCOS), two conditions affecting fertility. Salad greens, dairy products, calcium-enhanced foods, more vital plant-based milk, and dairy products all contain a lot of calcium.

4. Vitamin D

Vitamin D is necessary for maintaining calcium levels and is essential for fertility. This is impacted by egg quality, ovarian breaking point, and significant areas of strength and balance. Because of low skin synthesis and diminished sun exposure, numerous ladies above 40 might have lower vitamin D levels. Egg yolks, sleek fish, and set dairy items are ordinary wellsprings of vitamin D. Be that as it may, supplementation might be essential to keep up with ideal levels.

5. Omega-3 fatty acid

Omega-3 fatty acids, particularly EPA (eicosapentaenoic acid) and DHA (docosahexaenoic acid) have been linked to improved fertility outcomes. These vital fats further develop a course to the conceptive organs, lessen aggravation, and add to the creation of Reproductive ly designed substances. Omega-3 unsaturated fats can be found in walnuts, flaxseeds, chia seeds, and sleek fish like salmon and sardines.

6. Coenzyme 10 (CoQ10)

CoQ10 is an enhancement that forestalls infection and is fundamental for cell energy creation. Egg quality and fertility are affected by age-related decreases in CoQ10. In women over 40, supplementing with CoQ10 has increased egg quality and the likelihood of a successful conception. It is typically found in organ meats, fish, and plant-based foods like nuts and seeds.

7. Antioxidants

Reproductive cells are protected from oxidative pressure and DNA harm by the supplements zinc, selenium, nutrients C and E, and others that forestall disease. They assist in keeping up with the sperm and the egg. Natural citrus fruits, berries, dull mixed greens, nuts, seeds, whole grains, and vegetables all have anti-microbial properties. After talking with a specialist, cell support-rich nourishing enhancements might be a choice.

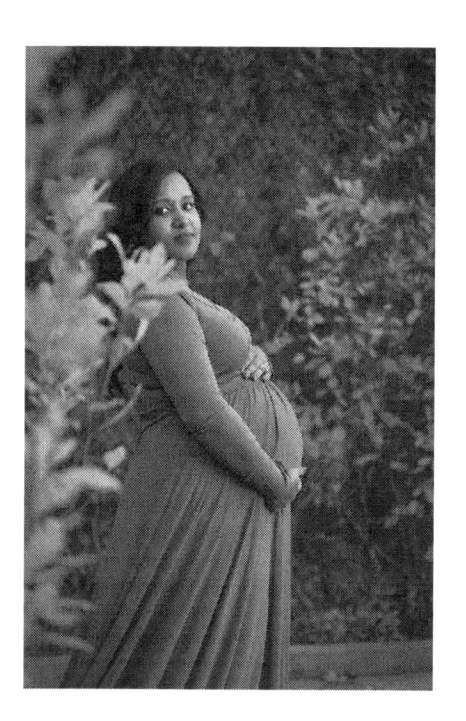

Chapter Two

Fertility Meal Plan Guidelines

Meal planning for fertility nutrition in women over 40 requires a thoughtful and balanced approach. While organizing your meal, you should be cautious and balanced.

You can give your body the nutrients it requires to assist Reproductive prosperity by knowing your caloric necessities, practicing portion control, ensuring a fair distribution of macronutrients, and prioritizing regular meals and snacks. Consult a registered dietitian with some experience in healthy food before creating a meal plan that meets your needs and goals.

Embrace these meal planning guidelines, empower yourself to nurture your fertility, and embrace motherhood's possibilities.

1. **Portion Control and Calorie Needs Management**

a. **Determine Your Calorie Needs:** As women advance in age, their metabolism commonly tones down, so they need fewer calories. A registered dietitian with some experience in healthy eating can determine your calorie needs based on age, weight, activity level, and overall health.

b. **Practice Portion Control:** It is essential to focus on portion sizes to remain aware of hormonal unity and maintain a healthy weight. It is possible to arrive at reasonable portions for various food groups by surveying cups, food scales, or visual cues. Attempt to eat different food groups that are nutrient-stacked on your plate while restricting how many calories are in food varieties.

2. **Balanced Macronutrient Distribution**

a. **Every meal should contain protein:** Protein is necessary for hormone production, egg quality, and conceptive prosperity. To encourage fertility, include lean protein sources like poultry, fish, vegetables, tofu, and Greek yogurt in every meal. For every supper, keep no pieces greater than 3 to 4 ounces.

b. **Choose Healthy Fats Only**: Healthy fats can help chemical blend and the assimilation of fat-solvent nutrients in your eating regimen. Excellent options include oily fish like salmon and sardines, avocados, olive oil, seeds, and nuts. To maintain equilibrium in major strength areas, use segment sizes.

c. **Indulge in Complex Carbs:** Your best options are whole grains, common foods, and vegetables with complex sugars. Vital vitamins and minerals, cell fortifications, fiber, and a constant energy supply are all packed into these. Refined and sugary starches should be avoided because they have the potential to alter blood sugar levels and lead to weight gain.

3. Importance of Regular Meals and Snacks

a. **Avoid skipping meals:** Consistency is fundamental in supporting your body for fertility. At the point when meals are skipped, chemical equilibrium can be upset, and glucose levels can vary. Aim for three balanced meals daily, with additional snacks if needed, to keep your energy levels stable and support overall reproductive health.

b. **Strategic Snacking:** Try not to overeat between meals. Choose nutritious options like Greek yogurt, raw nuts, fresh fruits, vegetable sticks with hummus as an addition, or new standard foods. Centre on portion sizes to make an effort not to eat such countless calories.

c. **Listen with Your Body:** Observe your body's signs to let you know when it is full and hungry. It would be best if you stopped eating when you were full. Eat when you are ravenous. The capacity to keep up with hormonal equilibrium, a Healthy relationship with food, and a good weight are among the many advantages of this mindful eating procedure.

CHAPTER THREE

The Fertility Diet Cookbook; Recipes Meal Plan and Meal Preparation

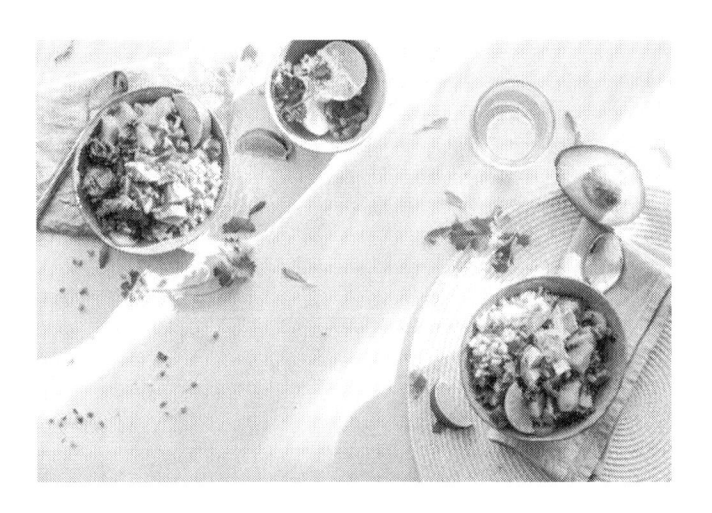

Embarking on a fertility journey is an extraordinary chapter in life. Regardless, providing your body with the appropriate food sources can make a big difference. A comprehensive guide, **"The Fertility Diet Cookbook,"** features flavorful recipes, a bespoke meal plan, and potent meal preparation tips. It is a joy for us to present it. Supplement-rich eats that help preparation, advance hormonal concordance, and further foster Reproductive prosperity are associated with this cookbook to empower female participation in the creation cycle. Plan for a culinary encounter that will maintain your body and soul while equivalently giving you a closer feel to enjoying life as a parent. Let's jump straight to the kitchen without wasting much of our time!

Day 1

Breakfast: Spinach and Mushroom Omelet

This healthy omelet of spinach and mushrooms is a great way to start your day. This recipe is flavorful and easy to plan, and its high centralization of fundamental supplements and minerals adds to its fertility. Spinach contains iron and folate, while mushrooms contain selenium and B vitamins that benefit reproductive health. Let's begin with the recipe to see how simple it is to prepare this filling meal.

Ingredients

Two large eggs
One cup of fresh spinach chopped finely
Half mushrooms are chopped finely
One tablespoon of olive oil

One-quarter teaspoon each of salt and pepper

Additional fixings:

- One grated cheese
- Avocado slices, or fresh herbs

Preparation:

1. Heat the olive oil to a medium temperature in a nonstick skillet.

2. The mushrooms should be cut in half and sautéed in a skillet for three to four minutes or until brown.

3. In the skillet, the chopped spinach should continue to cook for a few more minutes.

4. In a substitute bowl, beat the eggs thoroughly. Add pepper and salt to taste.

5. Pour the beaten eggs uniformly over the spinach and mushroom combination in the skillet.

6. Cooking time for the omelet should be two to three minutes or until the edges begin to set.

7. Lift the edges of the omelet gently with a spatula and incline the skillet so that any uncooked eggs can flow to the edges.

8. Right when the omelet is, for the most part, set and, at the same time, somewhat runny on top, meticulously package it in half with a spatula.

9. Cook another one to two minutes to ensure the omelet is perfectly cooked.

10. Add anything you like to the omelet on a plate, like avocado cuts, ground cheddar, or new flavors.

11. Serve hot, Healthy Spinach and Mushroom Omelet!

Meal Preparation Tips:

- You can prepare the spinach and mushrooms the prior night and store them independently in impenetrable holders in the fridge to save opportunity in the first part of the day.

- For meal preparation, store a larger batch of the spinach and mushroom mixture in the refrigerator. Just warm the blend in the first part of the day, beat the eggs, and immediately make an omelet.

- To personalize your omelet, add fertility-friendly ingredients like nutritional yeast, diced onions, or bell peppers for a cheesy flavor.

- Serve your spinach and mushroom omelet with whole-grain toast or fresh fruit for a healthy and balanced meal.

Note:

The spinach and mushroom omelet is a delicious and easy-to-include meal that helps with fertility and tastes good. This omelet provides a nutritious start to your day while supporting your fertility objectives. It is loaded up with nutrients, minerals, and other healthy goodness. You can have a feeding dinner that sorts you out for accomplishing ideal conceptive well-being by following the direct recipe and preparing early when functional.

Lunch: Grilled Salmon with Quinoa and Roasted Vegetables

Partake in a flavorful and nutrient-rich meal incorporating grilled salmon, quinoa, and simmered vegetables to further develop fertility sustenance. This combination is not only delicious, but it also provides essential nutrients that support reproductive health. Due to its abundance of vitamins and minerals, high-quality protein, and omega-3 fatty acids, this meal is an excellent choice for pregnant women. Let's examine the easy steps for making this filling dish and the recipe.

Ingredients:

- Two salmon fillets
- One cup of quinoa
- Two cups of water or vegetable broth

- Variety of vegetables like zucchini, bell peppers, and cherry tomatoes.
- One teaspoon of dried herbs, such as rosemary, oregano, or thyme
- Two tablespoons of olive oil
- Lemon wedges for serving
- Salt and pepper to taste

Preparation:

1. The grill should first be heated to a medium-high temperature.

2. Dry the salmon fillets with a paper towel after rinsing them in cold water. To taste, add salt and pepper.

3. Bring the water or vegetable broth to a boil in a saucepan. Reduce the heat to a simmer, add the quinoa, cover the pot, and cook for 15 to 20 minutes or until it is cooked through and fluffy.

4. While the quinoa cooks, prepare the vegetables. After being washed, cut them into bite-sized pieces.

5. Sprinkle olive oil, salt, pepper, and dried herbs on a baking sheet on top of the chopped vegetables. Equitably coat by throwing.

6. Cook the vegetables in the broiler for 15 to 20 minutes at 400 °F (200 °C) or until they are delicate and have started to caramelize.

7. Place the salmon fillets on the heated grill in the interim. The salmon should be cooked on each side for 4-5 minutes until it flakes easily and is thoroughly cooked.

8. Place a portion of cooked quinoa, grilled salmon, and roasted vegetables on your plate after everything has been prepared.

9. To give the salmon more flavor, press some new lemon juice over it.

10. Serve hot and relish your filling Quinoa-Simmered Vegetable Grilled Salmon!

Meal Preparation Tips:

- Marinate the salmon filets in lemon juice, olive oil, garlic, and spices to save time.

- Get ready more quinoa and cooked vegetables with the goal that you can have extras for another dinner or a fast lunch.

- To enhance the dish's freshness and flavor, add fresh herbs to the quinoa, such as dill or parsley.

- Assuming you favor different vegetables, substitute them for the ones referenced, contingent upon the season and your inclinations.

Note:

When trying to conceive, a flavorful, nutrient-dense meal like grilled salmon with quinoa and roasted vegetables is good for your reproductive health. This dish improves overall health thanks to its high protein content, high content of omega-3 fatty acids, and a wide variety of vegetables.

Follow the simple directions for this recipe to make a delicious meal that will fuel your body and help you achieve your fertility goals. Embrace the advantages of this healthy combination while enjoying the flavor of a meal that brings you one step closer to your goal of becoming a mother.

Dinner: Baked Chicken Breast with Sweet Potato and Broccoli

A delicious and nutritious meal with baked chicken breast, sweet potatoes, and broccoli will nourish your body and help you achieve fertility. In addition to providing plenty of protein, vitamins, and minerals beneficial to reproductive health, this combination provides a balanced supply of a wide range of nutrients. This meal is an extraordinary choice for ladies hoping to work on their fertility through sustenance due to its energetic varieties and filling flavors. Let's examine the easy steps for making this filling dish and the recipe.

Ingredients:

- Two medium sweet potatoes, diced and peeled
- Two boneless chicken breasts

- Two cups broccoli florets
- One teaspoon of garlic powder
- Two tablespoons of olive oil
- Paprika, One teaspoon
- Half a teaspoon of fresh lemon wedges for serving
- Salt and pepper to taste
- Dried thyme

Preparation:

1. Preheat the oven to 200°C (400°F).

2. Orchestrate the broccoli florets and diced potatoes on a baking sheet. Olive oil should be showered over the dish before adding salt, pepper, dried thyme, garlic powder, and paprika. To completely coat the vegetables, toss them in the seasoning.

3. Arrange the chicken breasts and seasoned vegetables on the same baking sheet. After drizzling the chicken breasts with olive oil, season them with salt, pepper, and any other seasonings you like.

4. Bake the baking sheet for 20 to 25 minutes until the chicken is cooked through and the sweet potatoes are soft and slightly golden.

5. Remove the baking sheet from the broiler, then, at that point, cut the chicken into serving-size pieces after it has rested for some time.

6. Divide the sweet potatoes, broccoli, and baked chicken breast among the plates.

7. Squeeze some fresh lemon juice over the chicken to add flavor and zest.

8. Partake in your hot, healthy dinner. Yam and broccoli with heated chicken bosom!

Meal Preparation Tips:

- Marinate the chicken bosoms for something like 30 minutes in a combination of olive oil, lemon juice, garlic, and spices for more flavor before baking.

- You can decide to season the chicken and vegetables any way you like. For more flavor and variety, consider incorporating spices like rosemary, chili powder, or cumin.

- Before baking the potatoes, you can cook them in the microwave for a couple of moments to save time. Cooking time will be reduced overall by doing this.

- For a vivid dish loaded with , go ahead and add other fertility cordial vegetables like asparagus, Brussels fledglings, or carrots, notwithstanding the potatoes and broccoli.

Note:
Surprisingly delicious and sustaining, heated chicken bosom with potatoes and broccoli advances fertility and general well-being. This blend offers indispensable nutrients for conceptive well-being and contains protein, nutrients, and minerals. You can partake in a nutritious and delicious dish that will fuel your body on your mission for fertility by complying with the clear recipe and meal fertility rules. This

well-balanced meal has many health benefits, tastes great, and is good for fertility.

Snack: Green Smoothie with Spinach and Berries

This vibrant and refreshing smoothie is loaded with nutrients from spinach and berries. Combining the goodness of leafy greens with the sweetness of berries makes this energizing recipe a delicious drink that helps with reproductive health. As you work toward becoming pregnant, this green smoothie, which is loaded with vitamins, minerals, and phytonutrients, is an excellent way to refuel your body. Let's examine the steps for making this reviving beverage and the recipe.

Ingredients:

- One cup of mixed berries, such as strawberries, blueberries, or raspberries, and one cup of fresh spinach.
- One tablespoon of a single ripe banana chia seeds
- One cup of unsweetened almond milk or any other plant-based milk

- Ice cubes
- A squeeze of lemon juice or a drizzle of honey for sweetness is optional.

Procedure:

1. Completely wash the spinach in cool water to dispose of any soil, debris, and jetsam.

2. Combine the chia seeds, almond milk, fresh spinach, mixed berries, and ripe banana in a blender.

3. For an additional burst of freshness, squeeze a bit of lemon juice over the top.

4. Add a few ice cubes if you'd like the smoothie to be colder and more energizing.

5. Utilize a fast blender to join every one of the fixings and make a smooth, rich consistency.

6. Adjust the smoothie's sweetness by tasting it and adding a little honey if necessary.

7. Drink the green smoothie straight from the glass or another container you brought with you.

Preparation Tips:

To save time in the morning or convenience while on the go, you can measure and prepare the spinach, berries, and chia seeds in advance and store them individually in freezer-safe bags. In the morning, take one out, add some almond milk to the blender, and start blending.

Try a variety of berry combinations to get more variety and antioxidant benefits. Depending on availability and personal preference, you can use fresh or frozen berries.

- Add some protein powder, almond margarine, flaxseeds, or other fertility-agreeable fixings to your green smoothie to make it your own. Flaxseeds will add more omega-3 unsaturated fats.

To make more servings, ponder multiplying the recipe. Before eating, any leftovers should be kept in an airtight container in the refrigerator for up to 24 hours.

Note:

The Green Smoothie with Spinach and Berries is refreshing and good for fertility. It can be eaten as a snack or as a healthy breakfast. This green smoothie, stacked with spinach, berries, and other healthy fixings, offers different pivotal supplements while advancing reproductive well-being. By following the straightforward recipe and making preparations whenever possible, you can enjoy a lively and reviving beverage that will energize your body on the path to improved fertility. Enjoy the vitality this green, healthy liquid will give you as you journey toward fertility.

Day 2

Breakfast: Overnight Chia Seed Pudding

You can start your day with a filling and delectable breakfast by indulging in Overnight Chia Seed Pudding. In addition to satisfying your palate, this delectable recipe offers vital nutrients that promote reproductive health. Chia seeds are an antioxidant, fiber, and omega-3 fatty acid powerhouse. You can have a wholesome breakfast in the morning by making this simple pudding the night before. Let's examine the recipe and straightforward cooking procedures for filling pudding.

Ingredients:

- One-fourth cup of chia seeds
- One cup of unsweetened almond milk or another plant-based milk
- One tablespoon of pure maple syrup or honey
- Half teas spoon of vanilla extract
- Fresh berries, sliced almonds, shredded coconut, or nut butter drizzle are optional toppings.

Preparation:

1. Combine the chia seeds, almond milk, vanilla extract, and pure maple syrup or honey in a bowl. To make sure the chia seeds are dispersed evenly, stir thoroughly.

2. Place the container in the fridge for at least 4-6 hours or overnight. Cover the container with a lid or plastic wrap. As a result, the chia seeds can absorb the liquid and take on the consistency of pudding.

3. Stir the chia seed mixture thoroughly in the morning to remove clumps and guarantee a smooth texture.

4. add your preferred toppings, such as fresh fruit, almond slices, coconut flakes, or a drizzle of nut butter for added flavor and texture.

5. Dish out your nutrient-rich Overnight Chia Seed Pudding chilled and enjoy!

Meal Preparation Tips:

- Add different flavors to your chia seed pudding to make it your taste. Add cocoa powder, cinnamon, or a tiny bit of matcha powder to improve the flavor.

- You can change the amount of sweetener if you like your pudding more sweet. Before chilling the mixture, taste it and, if needed, add more sweetener.

- Before serving, top the pudding with some ground flaxseeds or hemp seeds to boost fertility-friendly nutrients.

- For a quick and easy breakfast throughout the week, prepare a larger batch of chia seed pudding and divide it into individual portions. The pudding should be kept in the refrigerator in airtight containers.

- To change the flavor and texture of your chia seed pudding, try experimenting with various plant-based kinds of milk, such as coconut milk, oat milk, or soy milk.

Note:

An overnight chia seed pudding is a simple and filling breakfast option that promotes fertility and gives you a healthy start to the day. This pudding provides vital nutrients for reproductive health by including omega-3 fatty acids, fiber, and antioxidants. It's an enjoyable way to take advantage of the health benefits of chia seeds, thanks to their adaptable toppings and smooth, creamy texture. You can conveniently eat healthy food and advance your fertility goals by making this pudding the night before. As you start your fertility journey, embrace the simplicity and healthfulness of Overnight Chia Seed Pudding and savor every spoonful.

Lunch: chickpea salad with feta and avocado.

Boost your nutrition for fertility with a colorful and filling chickpea salad that includes creamy avocado and tangy feta cheese. This delicious recipe incorporates fertility-friendly ingredients that promote reproductive health and offer a light and satisfying meal. This salad is a fantastic option for women on their fertility journey because it contains plant-based protein, healthy fats, and various vitamins and minerals. Let's examine the recipe and the straightforward procedures for making this filling dish.

Ingredients:

- One can rinse and drain chickpeas
- One large diced ripe avocado
- One cup of halved cherry tomatoes
- Half cup diced cucumber
- One-quarter cup of finely chopped red onion
- Two tablespoons of fresh lemon juice.

- Two tablespoons of extra virgin olive oil
- Two tablespoons of chopped fresh parsley
- One quarter cup feta cheese, crumbled
- To taste, salt and pepper

Procedure:

1. To begin, combine the chickpeas, diced avocado, cherry tomatoes, cucumber, and red onion in a big bowl.

2. To make the dressing, combine the lemon juice, extra virgin olive oil, parsley that has been chopped, salt, and pepper in a small bowl.

3. Drizzle the dressing over the chickpea mixture and toss the ingredients to evenly coat them.

4. Add the feta cheese crumbles to the salad and give it a final gentle stir.

5. After tasting the salad, adjust the seasoning as desired by adding more salt, pepper, or lemon juice.

6. Let the salad marinate in the fridge for at least 15 to 20 minutes to allow the flavors to meld.

7. Just before serving, give the salad one last toss and top with some extra fresh parsley.

8. To enjoy your flavorful Chickpea Salad with Avocado and Feta, serve it chilled.

Meal Preparation Tips:

- You can use canned chickpeas rather than making them from scratch to save time. Thoroughly drain and rinse them to eliminate any extra sodium.

- Add extra vegetables to your salad, such as bell peppers, olives, or baby spinach, for more color and nutritional variety.

- For more crunch and nutrition, consider including a handful of toasted nuts or seeds, like pumpkin seeds or almonds.

- Before tossing the dressing with the salad, mash a small amount of the diced avocado and combine it with the lemon juice and olive oil for a creamier dressing.

- Remove the feta cheese or swap it out for a vegan cheese substitute if you prefer a vegan option.

Note:

A flavorful and nutrient-rich meal that promotes fertility and general well-being is chickpea salad with avocado and feta. This salad provides a balance of plant-based protein, healthy fats, and a range of vitamins and minerals thanks to the addition of chickpeas, avocado, and feta cheese. You can prepare a meal that will nourish your body on your quest for fertility by following the easy recipe and meal preparation advice. Enjoy the health advantages of this vibrant salad and the flavor of a filling, fertility-friendly meal.

Dinner: Brown rice and lentil curry for supper.

A flavorful lentil curry with nutritious brown rice will satisfy your palate and energize your body. In addition to offering a hearty and filling meal, this delectable recipe also uses fertility-friendly ingredients to support reproductive health. This curry is a fantastic option for women on their quest for fertility because it is stuffed with plant-based protein, fiber, and a variety of spices. Let's look at the instructions and discover how to make this wholesome dish.

Ingredients:

- One cup of rinsed and drained brown lentils
- One cup of brown rice
- One tablespoon of coconut oil
- One diced onion
- Three minced garlic cloves
- One tablespoon of grated fresh ginger
- One tablespoon curry powder.
- One teaspoon each of ground cumin, ground coriander, and turmeric
- One 14-ounce can of diced tomatoes
- One 14-ounce can of coconut milk
- Two cups of vegetable broth, salt, and pepper to taste. Chopped fresh cilantro.

Procedure:

1. Prepare the brown rice by following the directions on the package. Place aside.

2. Heat the coconut oil in a big pot over medium heat. When the onion is translucent, add it and continue to cook.

3. Fill the pot with the grated ginger and minced garlic. Cook until fragrant for one more minute.

4. Add the turmeric, cumin, coriander, and curry powder. To bring out the flavors of the spices, toast them for a minute.

5. Fill the pot with coconut milk, vegetable broth, diced tomatoes with juice, and lentils. To thoroughly combine all the ingredients, stir well.

6. Once the mixture has reached a rolling boil, turn the heat low and cover the pan. Allow the curry to simmer for approximately 25 to 30 minutes or until the lentils are cooked through and tender.

7. To taste, add salt and pepper to the curry. Adjust the seasoning by adding more curry powder or turmeric for a stronger taste.

8. Spoon the lentil curry over a bed of brown rice that has been cooked. Add fresh cilantro to the garnish for flavor and freshness.

9. Enjoy your filling and nourishing Brown Rice and Lentil Curry!

Meal Preparation Tips:

- You can sauté the spices in the coconut oil before including the onion, garlic, and ginger for a richer flavor. This will improve the curry's flavor and depth.

- Add more vegetables to the curry, such as diced carrots, bell peppers, or spinach, for added color, texture, and nutrients.

- Before serving, stir in a few tablespoons of coconut cream or plain Greek yogurt if you prefer a creamier curry.

- For a convenient and wholesome meal option throughout the week, prepare a larger batch of lentil curry and keep the leftovers in the refrigerator.

- For a filling and complete meal, serve the lentil curry with a side of naan bread or pita.

Note:

Brown rice and lentil curry is a filling and nourishing dish that promotes fertility and offers a delightful dining experience. This curry provides a balance of plant-based protein, fiber, and important nutrients thanks to the inclusion of lentils, flavorful spices, and wholesome brown rice. You can enjoy a tasty and nourishing meal that will fuel your body on your quest for fertility by following the easy recipe and meal preparation tips. Enjoy the flavor of a hearty, fertility-friendly dish while taking advantage of this comforting curry's health benefits.

Snacks: Greek yogurt parfait with granola and mixed berries.

Enjoy a delicious and nutrient-rich Greek yogurt parfait topped with various berries and crunchy granola. In addition to satisfying your cravings, this nutritious recipe offers vital nutrients for reproductive health. This parfait is a great option for women who are trying to get pregnant because it is full of protein, vitamins, and antioxidants. Let's look at the recipe and the straightforward procedures for making this delectable and fertility-friendly treat.

Ingredients:

- One cup of Greek yogurt.
- One tablespoon of optional honey
- Half cup granola (of your preferred type).
- One cup of mixed berries, including raspberries, blueberries, and strawberries.
- Optional garnish of fresh mint leaves

Preparation:

1. Thoroughly combine the Greek yogurt and optional honey in a small bowl. The honey gives the yogurt a hint of sweetness.

2. Place the ingredients in a clear glass or jar and begin layering. At the bottom, place a spoonful of Greek yogurt.

3. To give the yogurt a crunchy texture, scatter some granola on top.

4. Top the granola with a layer of mixed berries.

5. Continue layering until the desired quantity is reached or the ingredients are used up.

6. To add a splash of freshness and aesthetic appeal, top with a final dollop of Greek yogurt and a few fresh mint leaves.

7. Immediately serve the Greek yogurt parfait and savor it!

Meal Preparation Tips:

- To customize your parfait, use Greek yogurt with flavors like vanilla or berries—alternatively, top plain Greek yogurt with the honey or maple syrup you choose.

- To add variety and texture to your parfait, experiment with different kinds of granola, such as almond, coconut, or chocolate.

- You are welcome to combine and contrast the berries according to the season or easily accessible.

- Add extra toppings like a dusting of chia seeds, almond slices, or coconut flakes for added nutrition and crunch.

- You can make the parfait in advance by layering the ingredients in a carry-on container and chilling it overnight. This makes it possible for you to grab it on busy days as a quick and wholesome breakfast or snack.

Note:

Greek yogurt parfait with granola and mixed berries is a treat that promotes fertility and offers a delightful culinary experience. This parfait balances nutrients to energize your body with its combination of protein-rich Greek yogurt, fiber-rich granola, and antioxidant-rich mixed berries. You can enjoy a filling and flavorful treat that will fuel your body on your quest for fertility by following the straightforward recipe and meal preparation guidelines. Enjoy this layered parfait's health benefits and savor each spoonful as you promote the health of your reproductive system.

Day 3

Breakfast: Scrambled Eggs with Spinach and Tomato

A mouthwatering and nutritious way to start the day is with scrambled eggs topped with tomato and spinach. As well as fulfilling your sense of taste, this flavorful recipe offers fundamental nutrients that advance conceptive well-being. This breakfast option is a powerhouse of antioxidants, vitamins, and protein that will help you get pregnant. Adding spinach and tomatoes to the mixture will result in a breakfast of scrambled eggs that is flavorful and high in nutrients. Let's look at the recipe and the direct methods for making this filling breakfast.

Ingredients:

- Two large eggs.
- One medium tomato
- One tablespoon of additional virgin olive oil
- Salt and pepper to taste
- Optional topping: grated Parmesan or feta cheese.

Procedure:

1. Heat the olive oil in a nonstick skillet over medium heat.

2. Add the spinach and cook it in the skillet or until it wilts.

3. Add the diced tomato and cook for another minute or until the tomatoes soften slightly.

4. In a different bowl, thoroughly beat the eggs. Add salt and pepper to taste.

5. Combine the spinach and tomato mixture with the beaten eggs in the skillet.

6. Cook and scramble the eggs with the vegetables by gently stirring them.

7. Cook the scrambled eggs to your preference, whether you want them fully cooked or soft and moist.

8. Place the scrambled eggs on a plate and turn off the heat.

9. Finish the fried eggs with ground Parmesan cheddar or disintegrated feta cheddar to add flavor and smoothness to the fried eggs.

10. Serve the spinach-tomato-egg scrambled eggs warm to get your fill of vitamins and minerals!

Meal Preparation Tips:

- Sprinkle the scrambled eggs with a pinch of herbs or spices like paprika, basil, or oregano for a more flavorful dish.

- If you need a change from spinach, explore different greens like kale or Swiss chard.

- You are free to add vegetables, such as chime peppers or mushrooms, to your fried eggs to give them more tone and surface.

- For a heartier and all the more balanced breakfast, serve the fried eggs with entire wheat toast or an avocado side.

- The spinach and tomatoes can be washed, chopped, and diced in advance so they are ready for use in breakfast.

- To personalize your scrambled eggs, sprinkle nutritional yeast or hot sauce on top for an additional kick of flavor.

Note:

This breakfast option contains vegetables high in antioxidants and eggs, which are high in protein. It also provides essential nutrients for reproductive health. Because it has a simple recipe and can be made in various ways, you can enjoy a tasty and filling meal that helps your body get pregnant. Partake in each nibble of this nutritious breakfast and receive its well-being rewards as you start your day feeling recharged and invigorated.

Lunch: quinoa salad with grilled chicken and vegetables
This brilliant recipe incorporates fixings that are great for fertility and advanced reproductive well-being and offers a healthy, even diet. This salad is an incredible choice for ladies attempting to get pregnant because it is brimming with protein, fiber, and different nutrients and minerals. Let's examine the easy steps for making this filling dish and the recipe.

Ingredients:

- One cup of cooked quinoa, arranged per the bearings on the bundle.
- Two skinless, boneless bosoms of chicken
- One medium zucchini, cut across into cuts
- One red chime pepper, sliced
- One yellow chime pepper sliced

- One cup of cherry tomatoes halved
- Finely cleaved one-quarter cup red onion
- Two tablespoons of lemon juice
- Two tablespoons of additional virgin olive oil and two tablespoons of cleaved new basil.
- To taste, salt and pepper

Procedure:

1. The grill should first be heated to a medium-high temperature.

2. The chicken breasts should be seasoned with salt and pepper.

3. The chicken breasts should be cooked on each side for 6 to 8 minutes on the grill. After giving them a chance to rest, cut them into slight strips.

4. Brush the chime pepper and zucchini cuts with olive oil and season with salt and pepper.

5. Grill the ringer peppers and zucchini for 3 to 4 minutes on each side or until they are delicate and softly burned. Give

them time to cool down after removing them from the grill. From that point onward, cleave them up into reasonable pieces.

6. Join the cooked quinoa, grilled chicken, vegetables, cherry tomatoes, and red onion in a sizable bowl.

7. Mix the lemon juice, additional virgin olive oil, basil, salt, and pepper in a little bowl to make the dressing.

8. The dressing should cover the quinoa and chicken mixture. Throw everything together completely to cover.

9. Adjust the seasoning by adding more salt, pepper, or lemon juice after tasting the salad.

10. Allow the salad to marinate in the refrigerator for at least 15 to 20 minutes to allow the flavors to combine.

11. Prepare the plate of mixed greens before serving and top with new basil leaves.

12. Serve your savory Quinoa Salad with Grilled Chicken, Vegetables, and Quinoa Salad chilled to enjoy!

Meal Preparation Tips:

- Cook the quinoa the day before and grill the chicken breasts to save time when serving.

- For additional newness and nourishing assortment, add extra vegetables to the serving of mixed greens, like cucumber, avocado, or steamed broccoli.

- You could sprinkle some toasted pine nuts or slivered almonds for extra crunch and flavor.

- If you want to make this dish vegan, you can substitute grilled tofu or chickpeas, both of which are protein sources made from plants, in their place.

- To enhance the salad's flavor, incorporate your preferred herbs or spices, such as garlic, parsley, or mint, into the dressing.

Note:

Quinoa Salad with Grilled Chicken and Vegetables is a nutritious and flavorful dish that encourages fertility and provides a delightful culinary experience. Quinoa, grilled chicken, and various vegetables make this salad full of protein, fiber, and essential nutrients. You can partake in a delightful meal that will fuel your body on your journey for fertility by following the simple recipe and dinner prep guidance.

Dinner: Grilled shrimp with asparagus and quinoa.

Grilled shrimp, tender steamed asparagus and a bed of fluffy quinoa make a delicious and beneficial dish for fertility. In addition to satisfying the palate, this tasty dish provides essential nutrients for reproductive health. Due to its abundance of protein, vitamins, and minerals, this dish is an excellent choice for pregnant women. Let's examine the easy steps for making this delicious treat and the recipe.

Ingredients:

- One pound of peeled and deveined shrimp,
- One tablespoon of olive oil
- One teaspoon of paprika.
- Salt and pepper to taste,

- One cup of cooked quinoa cooked according to package directions
- One bunch of asparagus with the woody ends trimmed
- One lemon juice
- Two tablespoons of freshly chopped parsley

Procedure:

1. The grill should first be heated to a medium-high temperature.

2. Combine the olive oil, shrimp, paprika, garlic powder, salt, and pepper in a bowl. Throw completely to cover the shrimp equally.

3. Thread the seasoned shrimp onto skewers for easy grilling.

4. On the grill, cook the shrimp until they are opaque and pink, about two to three minutes per side. Take it off the Grill, then place it to the side.

5. Prepare the quinoa in the interim following the package's instructions. Set the cooked quinoa aside after being fluffed with a fork.

6. Steam the asparagus in a liner container for 5 to 7 minutes or until fresh yet delicate. Remove from the steamer and set aside.

7. Join the cooked quinoa, grilled shrimp, asparagus, lemon juice, and new parsley in a big bowl. Gently mix all of the ingredients.

8. You can adjust the dish by tasting it and adding more salt, pepper, or lemon juice if necessary.

9. To work on the taste, stand by a couple of moments before serving so the flavors can blend.

10. While still hot, Serve the grilled shrimp, quinoa, and steamed asparagus on separate plates.

Meal Preparation Tips:

- While the shrimp are marinating, add a squeeze of fresh lime juice or a pinch of chili flakes to give them more flavor.

- To enhance the dish's visual appeal and nutritional value, you are welcome to include additional grilled vegetables, such as zucchini or bell peppers.

- If you don't have a grill, cook the shrimp on the stovetop in a skillet or grill pan over medium-high heat for similar results.

- Try experimenting with herbs like cilantro or basil to give the dish a new flavor.

- Pair the grilled shrimp and quinoa dish with a fresh tomato salad or mixed greens for a well-rounded meal.

Note:

This delicious dish of grilled shrimp, quinoa, and steamed asparagus is good for fertility and makes a good meal. With its succulent grilled shrimp, fluffy quinoa, and vibrant steamed asparagus, this dish balances protein, fiber, and important nutrients. By adhering to the straightforward instructions for the recipe and the meal preparation, you can savor a nutritious meal that will help you achieve fertility. Take advantage of the numerous benefits of this delicious dish while you savor each bite and nourish your reproductive health.

Snack: carrot sticks and hummus

This is a mouthwatering combination that will satisfy your snacking itch. In addition to providing a satisfying crunch, this straightforward but filling snack provides nutrients essential for reproductive health. Because it contains a lot of fiber, vitamins, and good fats, this carrot and hummus combination is a great option for women trying to conceive.

Let's look at the ingredients and how to make this tasty snack good for fertility.

Ingredients:
- Freshly washed and peeled carrots
- Homemade or store-bought hummus
- Paprika, chopped fresh parsley, or extra virgin olive oil as optional garnishes.

Preparation:
1. After thoroughly washing the carrots, peel them.

2. Slice the carrots into sticks of the desired length and thickness to make them easy to dip into the hummus.

3. The carrot sticks can be served in individual snack containers or on a platter.

4. Place a liberal spot of hummus close to the carrot sticks in a different serving bowl.

5. Optionally top the hummus with chopped fresh parsley or a pinch of paprika to enhance its flavor and appearance.

6. Drizzle some olive oil on the hummus for a smoother texture and enhanced flavor.

7. Quickly serve the hummus and carrot sticks and appreciate!

Feel free to use various carrots in various colors, such as yellow, orange, or purple, to enhance the snack's visual appeal.

Preparation Tips:

- To change up your determination of tidbits, attempt hummus in flavors like broiled red pepper, garlic, or lemon.

- Add a few seeds, like sesame or pumpkin, to the hummus for additional crunch and sustenance to work on the wholesome profile.

- Try dipping cucumber slices, bell pepper strips, or celery sticks in the hummus alongside the carrot sticks for a flavorful alternative.

- Make your own hummus with chickpeas, tahini, lemon squeeze, and flavors for a more individualized and healthy choice.

Note:

Carrot sticks with hummus are a delicious and sound bite that advances fertility. This site offers an equilibrium of supplements fundamental for conceptive well-being because it blends fiber-rich carrots and protein-rich hummus. By following the straightforward preparation steps and incorporating your preferred hummus flavors and toppings, you can enjoy a nutritious and flavorful snack that will fuel your body in your quest for fertility. Acknowledge the upsides of this speedy and sound choice, and partake in each significant piece as you support your reproductive well-being.

Day 4:

Breakfast: Berry Smoothie Bowl with Almond Margarine and Granola.

Get your day going with a berry smoothie bowl with velvety almond spread and crunchy granola for an energetic day. As well as fulfilling your sense of taste, this refreshing recipe offers fundamental supplements for reproductive well-being. Because it is loaded with healthy fats, fiber, and antioxidants, this smoothie bowl is an excellent choice for women trying to conceive. Learn how to make this tasty and filling breakfast by following the recipe.

Ingredients:

- One cup of strawberries, blueberries, and raspberries, either fresh or frozen.
- A half cup of almond milk (or another kind of milk)
- One teaspoon of almond butter.
- Granola, chia seeds, shredded coconut, and thinly sliced fresh fruit are optional toppings.

Preparation:

1. Combine the mixed berries, frozen banana, almond milk, and almond butter in a blender.

2. Blend the combination until it is smooth and creamy. If you need more almond milk to get the right consistency, add it.

3. The berry smoothie mixture should be put in a bowl.

4. Sliced fresh berries, chia seeds, shredded coconut, and a generous amount of granola are some garnishes that can be added to the smoothie bowl to give it more texture and flavor.

5. Serve the Berry Smoothie Bowl immediately and enjoy your nutrient-packed breakfast!

Meal Preparation Tips:

Investigate all the possibilities for different berry blends to suit your preferences.

Add spinach or kale to the smoothie to increase vitamins and minerals.

Mix in your preferred superfoods, such as sliced almonds, pumpkin seeds, or goji berries, to personalize your toppings.

Drizzle a little honey or maple syrup on top to add even more sweetness to the smoothie bowl.

Set up the smoothie ingredients the night before and keep them in individual holders in the cooler for a quick and convenient breakfast.

Get creative with the presentation and arrange the toppings to make them look good to make your smoothie bowl even more enticing.

Note:

The berry smoothie bowl with almond butter and granola is a delicious and nourishing breakfast that promotes conception and gives you a refreshing start to the day. This smoothie bowl offers a balance of vitamins, minerals, and good fats thanks to its combination of cellular-reinforcing berries, velvety almond spread, and crunchy granola. By following the simple recipe and meal preparation instructions, you can enjoy a nourishing and delicious meal that will fuel your body on your quest for fertility. Enjoy the advantages of this vibrant and flavorful smoothie bowl and savor each spoonful as you nourish your reproductive health.

Lunch: Roasted vegetable and goat cheese quiche

This is a delectable dish that satisfies the taste buds and supplies vital nutrients for reproductive health. Enjoy the tantalizing flavors of a Quiche with Goat Cheese and Roasted Vegetables. Roasted vegetables and creamy goat cheese are placed on top of the flaky crust of this delectable quiche. Because it contains a lot of protein, vitamins, and minerals, this recipe is a great choice for women who are trying to get pregnant. Before diving into the recipe, explore the steps involved in preparing this brilliant and rich cordial dish.

Ingredients:

- One pie crust, either homemade or from a store

- One cup of mixed roasted vegetables, including bell peppers, zucchini, and onions.
- Four large eggs
- One cup of milk, either vegan or dairy
- Four oz. crumbled goat cheese
- Fresh herbs for garnish (optional)
- salt and pepper to taste

Procedure:

1. Set the oven to 375°F (190°C).

2. Set aside the pie crust prepared in a pie dish.

3. Thoroughly combine the milk, eggs, salt, and pepper in a bowl.

4. Distribute the cooked vegetables blended in an even layer over the pie crust's bottom.

5. Ensure that the egg and milk mixture is evenly distributed over the vegetables.

6. Sprinkle the goat cheddar crumbles on the quiche.

7. Carefully transfer the quiche to the preheated broiler and cook for 30-35 minutes until the quiche is set and the top is a brilliant golden brown.

8. After taking the quiche out of the oven, let it cool.

9. If desired, add fresh herbs like basil or parsley as a garnish before serving the dish.

10. After cutting the Quiche with Roasted Vegetables and Goat Cheese into wedges, serve it warm or at room temperature.

Meal Preparation Tips:

- To save time, use pre-broiled vegetables, prepare them, and store them in the refrigerator until needed.

- Explore different options for different vegetable combinations based on your preferences and what's in season.

- Instead of making a pie crust, you can make a quiche without one by pouring the egg mixture into a greased pie dish.

- Integrate toppings like sun-dried tomatoes, caramelized onions, or fresh spinach to add additional flavors and textures.

- For a well-balanced and supplemental thick dinner, serve the quiche with a side plate of mixed greens or steamed vegetables.

Note:

Roasted Vegetable and Goat Cheese Quiche is a savory delight that supports fertility and provides a satisfying and flavorful dining experience. This quiche provides the right balance of nutrients needed for regenerative health with its combination of broiled vegetables, velvety goat cheddar, and a delicate outer layer. By following the simple recipe and meal preparation instructions, you can enjoy a delicious dish that promotes fertility and nourishes your body during your attempt to conceive. Enjoy every bite of this tantalizing quiche while promoting the health of your reproductive system.

Dinner: Baked Cod with Lemon-Dill Sauce, Quinoa, and Roasted Brussels Sprouts

Enjoy a delicious and healthy dinner of prepared cod, served with fluffy quinoa and roasted Brussels sprouts. The dish is finished with a zesty lemon-dill sauce. This delicious combination offers essential nutrients for reproductive health and tantalizes your taste buds. This recipe is a fantastic choice for women trying to get pregnant because it is packed with vitamins, protein, and omega-3 fatty acids. How about we look into the recipe and prepare this delectable and fruitful meal?

Ingredients:

- Four cod fillets
- Two tablespoons of lemon juice
- Two teaspoons of lemon zest,
- Two tablespoons of fresh chopped dill
- Salt and pepper to taste
- One cup of rinsed quinoa
- Two cups of water or vegetable broth
- One pound of halved Brussels sprouts

- Two tablespoons of olive oil.

Procedure:

1. You should preheat your oven to 200°C (400°F).

2. Combine the lemon juice, zing, fresh dill, salt, and pepper in a small bowl to create the Lemon-Dill Sauce. Set apart.

3. After seasoning the cod filets with salt and pepper, place them on a baking sheet lined with parchment paper.

4. Divide the remaining Lemon-Dill Sauce in half and serve it alongside the cod fillets.

5. Bake the cod for 12 to 15 minutes in a preheated oven or until it flakes easily and is thoroughly cooked.

6. While the cod bakes, mix the quinoa with water or vegetable broth in a saucepan. Once the quinoa is fluffy and the entire liquid has been absorbed, simmer it for 15-20 minutes, then bring it to a boil.

7. The Brussels sprouts should be mixed with olive oil, salt, and pepper. Spread them on a baking sheet, then broil them for 20 to 25 minutes or until tender and slightly caramelized.

8. After cooking, divide the cod, quinoa, and grilled Brussels sprouts among serving plates.

9. Pour the rest of the lemon-dill sauce over the cod fillets.

10. Immediately serve the cooked cod with quinoa, grilled Brussels sprouts, and a lemon-dill sauce so everyone can enjoy your delicious and wholesome dinner.

Meal Preparation Tips:

- Pick brand-new, top-notch cod filets for the best flavor and texture when preparing a meal.

- For a crispier texture, finish broiling the cod for a few minutes.

- For a pleasant touch, adjust the Lemon-Dill Sauce by incorporating some minced garlic or honey.

- Quinoa will taste better when cooked in vegetable broth or adding herbs and spices to the cooking liquid.

- If you prefer a different side dish, experiment with different cooking methods with other simmered vegetables like carrots, yams, or asparagus.

Note:

You can get pregnant while indulging your taste bud by eating baked cod with lemon-dill sauce, quinoa, and roasted Brussels sprouts. Thanks to the omega-3-rich cod, zingy Lemon-Dill Sauce, protein-rich quinoa, and nutrient-dense Brussels sprouts, this meal offers a balanced supply of essential nutrients for reproductive health. You can enjoy a tasty and fertility-friendly dinner that aids your body in becoming pregnant by following the simple recipe and meal preparation advice. Enjoy every bite of this flavorful meal while supporting your reproductive health.

Snack: Slices of cucumber with tzatziki sauce.

A Refreshing and Healthful Snack for Women Over 40.

Slices of cucumber with tzatziki sauce make a tasty and hydrating snack that complements a fertility diet for women over 40. They are hydrating, crunchy, and nutrient-rich. This simple but flavorful mixture offers a delightful balance of tastes, textures, and essential nutrients. Let's discuss the ingredients, how to prepare it, and the benefits of including this nutritious treat in your quest for fertility.

Ingredients:
- One large, thinly sliced cucumber,
- One cup of Greek yogurt,
- Half a cup of grated cucumber,
- One minced garlic clove,
- One tablespoon of extra-virgin olive oil,
- One tablespoon of fresh lemon juice,
- One tablespoon of chopped fresh dill,
- Salt and pepper to taste.

Procedure:

1. First, make the tzatziki sauce. Combine Greek yogurt, grated cucumber, minced garlic, fresh lemon juice, extra virgin olive oil, and chopped dill in a bowl. The ingredients should be thoroughly mixed together.

2. To taste, You only need to season the tzatziki sauce with salt and pepper. As necessary, season the food.

3. The cucumber should then be washed and cut into thin rounds. You can strip the cucumber or leave the skin intact, depending on your preference.

4. Arrange the cucumber slices on individual plates or a serving platter.

5. Cover each cucumber cut with the tasty tzatziki sauce by liberally spooning it over the cucumber slices.

6. Sprinkle fresh dill on top to add decoration and more locally grown freshness.

7. Serve the tzatziki sauce and cucumber slices immediately and savor this cooling snack.

Meal Preparation Tips:

- To make a thicker tzatziki sauce, strain the Greek yogurt and grated cucumber through a fine-mesh sieve or cheesecloth to remove any extra moisture.

- For flavor, try experimenting with extra herbs and spices like cumin, mint, or parsley.

- Serve the cold cucumber slices and tzatziki sauce to make them even more cooling on hot summer days.

- To make your snack special, serve the cucumber slices with whole-grain crackers, pita bread, or as a side dish with a meal.

Note:

Cucumber slices with tzatziki sauce offer a delectable fusion of tastes, textures, and nourishing qualities. This energizing snack also offers a hydrating crunch and contains the probiotics of Greek yogurt, the goodness of fresh cucumber, and essential nutrients. This quick, delectable snack can help you eat a healthy, balanced diet while adding variety to your fertility meal plan. Enjoy the crispness of the cucumber and the creamy tang of the tzatziki sauce in this reviving snack that promotes conception. We're happy to hear that you're fertile and healthy!

Day 5:

Breakfast: Burrito made with whole wheat tortilla

Start your day with a filling Veggie Breakfast Burrito made with whole wheat tortilla and stuffed with flavorful spices and nutritious vegetables. This delicious and filling breakfast option is quick and easy to prepare and provides the essential ingredients for a healthy start to the day. This veggie breakfast burrito is a fantastic choice for women undergoing fertility because it is packed with fiber, nutrients, and cell reinforcements. Let's start with the recipe to discover how to prepare this nourishing breakfast beneficial for conception.

Ingredients:
- Four large eggs
- Four whole-wheat tortillas

- A cup of chopped mixed vegetables (such as bell peppers, onions, spinach, and mushrooms)
- Half a teaspoon of ground cumin
- Half a teaspoon of paprika
- Salt and pepper to taste
- Optional salsa, avocado slices, cheese crumbles, and fresh cilantro

Procedure:

1. Before heating a nonstick skillet to medium heat, lightly coat it with cooking spray or olive oil.

2. In a bowl, thoroughly whisk the eggs. Add to taste the paprika, ground cumin, salt, and pepper. Set aside.

3. The blended vegetables cut into pieces should be added to the skillet and sautéed for a few seconds until soft.

4. The skillet should be filled with vegetables and the beaten eggs. The eggs should be cooked through and scrambled, stirring event ally.

5. The whole wheat tortillas should be malleable when heated briefly in the microwave or a different skillet.

6. Each tortilla should have the vegetable mixture and scrambled eggs in the center.

7. If desired, add your preferred garnishes, such as salsa, avocado slices, crumbled cheddar, or fresh cilantro.

8. Fold the tortilla's sides over the filling and roll it up tightly to create a burrito.

9. For each tortilla, repeat the cycle.

10. Serve the Veggie Breakfast Burritos warm, and enjoy a delicious and healthy start to your day.

Meal Preparation Tips:

- To change the flavor and texture of your Veggie Breakfast Burrito, add extra fixings like dark beans, diced tomatoes, or jalapenos.

- Any vegetables you prefer or have in your refrigerator may be used. Try various combinations to keep it interesting.

- Mix some chili powder or hot sauce into the egg mixture for a spicier burrito before cooking.

- Add a few tablespoons of cooked quinoa or tofu to the vegetable and egg mixture to boost the amount of protein.

- For a quick and simple breakfast option on hectic mornings, prepare a batch of veggie breakfast burritos in advance and freeze each one separately.

Note:

The Veggie Breakfast Burrito with Whole Wheat Tortilla is a healthy and energizing way to start your day while supporting your fertility journey. Thanks to scrambled eggs, nutrient-dense vegetables, and whole wheat tortillas, this breakfast offers a balanced intake of essential nutrients for reproductive health. You can participate in a delicious and fertility cordial meal that supports your body and keeps you satisfied throughout the morning by adhering to the basic recipe and breakfast burrito planning guidelines. Enjoy this flavorful and nourishing breakfast while promoting your reproductive health.

Lunch: Grilled chicken Caesar salad with whole-grain Croutons

Enjoy a delicious and nutritious grilled chicken Caesar salad with whole grain bread garnishes for a nutritious, nutrient-rich dinner. This traditional salad is elevated by grilled chicken, crisp romaine lettuce, and whole grain croutons, making it a delicious and nourishing choice for women trying to improve their reproductive health. This salad provides a well-balanced blend of supplements packed with protein, fiber, nutrients, and minerals. Why don't we look into the recipe and prepare for this delicious and convivial meal?

Ingredients:

- One head of romaine lettuce that has been washed and chopped
- One cup whole grain croutons

- One-quarter cup grated Parmesan cheese, homemade or pre-made Caesar dressing,
- Salt and pepper to taste
- An optional garnish of sliced red onions, cucumbers, and cherry tomatoes

Procedure:

1. The grill or pan should be heated to a medium-high setting.

2. Add salt and pepper to the chicken breasts before serving.

3. Grill the chicken breasts on each side for 6 to 8 minutes or until they reach an internal temperature of 165°F (74°C). Remove the intensity and give them a brief moment to rest before cutting.

4. Set up the plate of mixed greens while the chicken grills by combining the chopped romaine lettuce, whole grain bread toppings, and ground Parmesan cheddar in a sizable mixing bowl.

5. Mix the Caesar dressing well with the salad ingredients to coat them evenly. As you like, increase the amount of dressing from a small starting point.

6. The chicken breasts should be thinly sliced after grilling.

7. Place the mixed greens on individual plates or a serving platter after dressing.

8. Add the cut grilled chicken to the serving of mixed greens.

9. Add thinly sliced red onions, cherry tomatoes, or cucumbers to the salad for additional flavor and freshness.

10. Enjoy the delicious fusion of flavors and surfaces by immediately serving the grilled chicken Caesar salad with whole grain bread garnishes.

Meal Preparation Tips:

- Cut whole grain bread into reduced-down healthy shapes and toss them with olive oil, garlic powder, and a little salt to make hand-crafted bread garnishes.

In a preheated oven, bake them for 10 to 15 minutes at 375°F (190°C) to make them crisp.

- To reduce the calorie count while maintaining the dressing's rich texture and tart flavor, use Greek yogurt or a mixture of Greek yogurt and mayonnaise.

- Increase the nutrient content of a serving of mixed greens by including extra vegetables like roasted red peppers, steamed asparagus, or artichoke hearts.

- If you prefer a vegetarian version, swap the grilled chicken for grilled tofu or chickpeas for a plant-based protein alternative.

Note:

Grilled chicken, Caesar salad with whole grain bread garnishes is a wholesome and satisfying meal that supports your fertility goals while enticing your taste buds. This salad, which includes grilled chicken, crisp romaine lettuce, whole grain croutons, and tangy Caesar dressing, offers a full range of nutrients that support reproductive health. Following the simple recipe and salad preparation instructions, you can enjoy a delicious, fertility-friendly meal nourishing your body as you navigate infertility. Enjoy every bite of this flavorful and nutrient-rich salad while promoting the health of your reproductive system.

Dinner: Baked Turkey Meatballs with Marinara Sauce, Whole Wheat Pasta, and Steamed Broccoli

Enjoy the heavenliness of Prepared Turkey Meatballs with Marinara Sauce, Whole Wheat Pasta, and Steamed Broccoli. This nutritious and delectable meal satisfies your cravings and provides essential nutrients for your fertility. This filling dish is completed with whole wheat pasta, lean turkey meatballs baked to perfection, a hearty marinara sauce, and nutrient-rich steamed broccoli. This dinner option supports your conceptual well-being while providing a wonderful flavor medley because it is packed with protein, fiber, nutrients, and minerals. Let's examine the ingredients and preparation of this meal that promotes fertility.

Ingredients:

For the turkey meatballs: The marinara sauce consists of:
- One pound lean ground turkey
- Half cup whole wheat breadcrumbs
- One-quarter cup of grated Parmesan cheese
- One quarter finely chopped fresh parsley
- One-quarter cup finely chopped onion
- Two minced cloves of garlic
- One large egg,
- Salt and pepper to taste.
- Two cups of homemade or locally sourced tomato puree
- Two minced garlic cloves
- Half teaspoon oregano, dried
- One-half teaspoon of dried basil
- To taste, salt and pepper

For the broccoli and pasta:
- A complete wheat pasta of your choice.
- Fresh florets of broccoli

Procedure:

1. You should preheat your oven to 200°C (400°F).

2. Ground turkey, whole wheat breadcrumbs, grated Parmesan cheese, egg, chopped parsley, chopped onion, minced garlic, dried oregano, dried basil, salt, and pepper are all included in this recipe for the turkey meatballs. Combine all the turkey meatballs ingredients in a large mixing bowl. Ensure that all of the ingredients are well combined.

3. Create desired-sized meatballs from the mixture, then place them on a baking sheet lined with parchment paper.

4. The turkey meatballs should be cooked through and sautéed on the outside after 20 to 25 minutes under the preheated broiler.

5. While the meatballs are baking, make the marinara sauce. The pureed tomatoes, minced garlic, dried oregano, dried basil, salt, and pepper should all be combined in a pan. The sauce should simmer on low heat for 10 to 15 minutes, stirring event ally.

6. As directed on the package, the whole wheat pasta must be cooked until it's al dente. Channel, then store.

7. Broccoli florets must be steamed until tender but still have a bright green color. Set aside.

8. Combine the marinara sauce and cooked whole wheat pasta in a sizable serving bowl to coat the pasta.

9. Pasta should be topped with baked turkey meatballs.

10. Enjoy this delicious and healthy dinner that supports your fat-burning process by serving the heated turkey meatballs with marinara sauce, whole wheat pasta, and steamed broccoli.

Meal Preparation Tips:

- To enhance the flavor of the turkey meatball mixture, add extra spices and flavors like dried thyme, rosemary, or red pepper chips.

- If you'd prefer a meatless option, you can use veggie lover meatballs made from ingredients like lentils, quinoa, or chickpeas instead of the turkey meatballs.

- Feel free to change the marinara sauce by including sautéed onions, bell peppers, or mushrooms for more flavor and texture.

- Drizzle some olive oil to make it a complete meal—snack: blended berries with whipped cream.

Snack: Mixed Berries with Whipped Cream

A serving of Blended Berries with Whipped Cream is a revitalizing and nutrient-rich pastry that adds a touch of pleasantness to your fertility process. Savor the wonderful combination of sweet and tart flavors with a serving. With a light, fluffy whipped cream topping, the natural sweetness of mixed berries is brought to life in this elegant dessert. Thanks to its abundant antioxidants, vitamins, and minerals, this dessert satisfies your sweet tooth and provides essential nutrients for reproductive health. Let's get started with the recipe and instructions for making this treat that promotes fertility.

Ingredients:

- Blackberries
- Blueberries
- strawberries, and other fresh berries
- One cup of heavy whipping cream
- Two tablespoons powdered sugar (adjust to taste)
- One teaspoon of vanilla extract.

Procedure:

1. After the fresh berries have been thoroughly washed in cold water, dry them using a paper towel. If desired, slice the strawberries after removing any leaves or stems.

2. Combine the powdered sugar, heavy whipping cream, and vanilla extract in a sizable mixing bowl.

3. Use an electric or whisk mixer to gently whisk the cream mixture into soft peaks. If you whip it too much, it might turn into butter.

4. When the whipped cream has reached the ideal consistency, taste it and, if necessary, adjust the sweetness by adding more powdered sugar. Set aside.

5. Layer the blended berries in serving bowls or glasses. You can alternate between different berries or develop a clever strategy utilizing just one kind of berry.

6. Add a generous dollop of whipped cream on top of the mixed berries.

7. You could garnish with a mint leaf or a sprinkle of powdered sugar for an extra touch of elegance.

8. Right away, serve the Mixed Berries with Whipped Cream so the flavors can meld together for a delectable dessert.

Preparation Tips:

- Look into different options for berry combinations to create a unique blend. Seasonal berries like currants or cranberries can be added for more variety.

- Greek yogurt or coconut cream can be used instead of heavy whipping cream to create a lighter, dairy-free whipped topping.

- To improve the flavor of the mixed berries, squeeze in some fresh lemon juice or sprinkle on a little cinnamon before adding the whipped cream.

- To add texture to the whipped cream, think about strewing toasted nuts like sliced almonds or crushed pistachios.

- If you prefer a make-ahead option, prepare the whipped cream separately and keep it in the refrigerator until serving. To maintain the freshness of the berries, gather the sweetness before you enjoy it.

Note:

Blended berries with whipped cream offer a reviving and nutrient-rich treatment option for your fertility process. This dessert provides a wonderful and satisfying end to your meal because it is filled with vibrant varieties and kinds of grouped berries and is joined with light and vaporous whipped cream. Enjoy the berries' natural pleasantness and cell-reinforcing rich decency while indulging in the velvety and extravagant whipped cream. Enjoy this dessert that promotes fertility while nourishing your body and reproductive system. Savor each spoonful.

Day 6

Breakfast: Avocado Toast with Smoked Salmon and Tomato

Avocado Toast with Smoked Salmon and Tomato is a flavorful and healthy way to start the day. The perfect balance of creamy avocado, salty smoked salmon, and juicy tomato slices in this delectable breakfast dish makes for a satisfying, healthy meal for women over 40. This avocado toast variation is a great option to support your fertility and general well-being because it is loaded with protein, healthy fats, and necessary nutrients. Let's explore this delicious breakfast option's recipe, preparation advice, and wonderful advantages.

Ingredients:

- Two slices of toasted whole-grain bread
- One mature avocado
- Half a lemon's juice
- Four ounces of smoked salmon - Salt and pepper to taste
- One sliced tomato
- Fresh dill or chives as an optional garnish

Procedure:

1. Cut the avocado in half, scoop out the flesh into a small bowl, and discard the pit.

2. Use a fork to mash the avocado to the desired consistency—salt, pepper, and lemon juice to taste. Mix thoroughly.

3. Evenly cover the toasted slices of whole grain bread with the mashed avocado.

4. Arrange the smoked salmon in an even layer on the avocado.

5. Place the tomatoes in slices over the smoked salmon.

6. To add a finishing touch, garnish the dish with fresh chives or dill for an additional flavor and aesthetic appeal.

7. Serve your avocado toast with smoked salmon, tomato, and other toppings immediately to enjoy the ideal fusion of flavors and textures.

Meal Preparation Tips:

Use ripe avocados that give light pressure when squeezed for the creamiest and most flavorful mashed avocado.

To keep the mashed avocado from browning and add a zesty tang, squeeze some fresh lemon juice.

Tailor the seasoning to your personal preferences. Consider including more herbs, spices, or a dash of hot sauce for an extra kick.

Choose whole grain bread to increase fiber content and give your avocado toast a healthier base.

For more flavor and variety, experiment with tomato varieties, such as heirloom or cherry tomatoes.

Replace the smoked salmon with thinly sliced cucumber or a sprinkle of nutritional yeast for a cheesy flavor if you're vegan.

You can further customize your avocado toast by sprinkling on garnishes like micro greens, red onion slices, or a drizzle of balsamic glaze.

Note:

For women over 40, avocado toast with smoked salmon and tomato is a delicious and filling breakfast option. This toast offers a well-balanced mix of healthy fats, protein, and important nutrients with its creamy avocado, savory smoked salmon, and refreshing tomato slices. With this delicious breakfast, you can give your body the nutrients it needs to support fertility. Enjoy the delicious flavors and take advantage of the many advantages of this delicious Avocado Toast creation. Good morning, and enjoy a wonderful start to your day!

Lunch: Quinoa Stuffed Bell Peppers with Ground Turkey:

Enjoy the hearty and well-rounded Quinoa Stuffed Bell Peppers with Ground Turkey, a dish that combines the goodness of quinoa with lean ground turkey and vibrant bell peppers. This delicious dish satisfies your palate and gives older women the nutrients they need to support their fertility and general health. This recipe is a great addition to your fertility diet because it contains protein, fiber, vitamins, and minerals. Let's look at this wholesome dish's ingredients, preparation advice, and amazing advantages.

Ingredients:

- Four large, any-color bell peppers
- One cup of cooked quinoa, one pound of lean ground turkey.
- One small onion, finely chopped
- Two cloves of minced garlic
- One teaspoon of dried oregano
- Half teaspoon paprika

- One teaspoon of ground cumin
- Half a teaspoon of salt
- One-quarter teaspoon of black pepper
- One cup of diced tomatoes, either fresh or in a can.
- Optional: Half a cup of shredded mozzarella cheese
- Freshly chopped parsley or cilantro (for garnish)

Procedure:

1. Set your oven to 375°F (190°C) for preparation.

2. Cut off the bell peppers' tops and scoop out the seeds and membranes. The peppers should be rinsed before storing.

3. Heat some olive oil in a big skillet over medium heat. Add the minced garlic and onion and sauté until fragrant and translucent.

4. Using a wooden spoon, break up the ground turkey into smaller pieces as it cooks in the skillet, browning it as it cooks.

5. Add the paprika, ground cumin, dried oregano, salt, and black pepper. To allow the flavors to meld, cook for one more minute.

6. Combine everything in the skillet after adding the cooked quinoa and diced tomatoes. Once everything is well combined, cook for a few more minutes.

7. Spoon the quinoa and ground turkey mixture into each bell pepper, packing it down firmly but gently.

8. Set the bell peppers stuffed in a baking dish and cover them with aluminum foil.

9. Bake for about 30 minutes in the preheated oven. After that, remove the foil and, if preferred, cover the peppers' tops with shredded mozzarella cheese. Bake the dish for 10 minutes, uncovered, or until the cheese is melted and bubbling.

10. Take the stuffed bell peppers out of the oven and set them aside to cool. Add fresh cilantro or parsley as a garnish.

11. As a main filling dish, serve the quinoa-stuffed bell peppers with ground turkey and enjoy the flavors and nutrients it offers.

Preparation Tips:

- Feel free to add other vegetables, such as zucchini, mushrooms, or spinach, to the filling to add extra flavor and nutrition.

- Replace the ground turkey in the recipe with vegetarian options like lentils, black beans, or chickpeas.

- For the best texture and flavor, choose firm, vibrantly colored bell peppers.

- Before incorporating the quinoa into the filling mixture, cook it as directed on the package.

- Add red pepper flakes or hot sauce to the filling mixture if you like hotter food.

- The stuffed peppers can also be made ahead of time and stored in the refrigerator until you're ready to bake them.

Note:

Ground turkey and quinoa stuffed bell peppers are tasty and healthy dishes that add variety and nutrition to your fertility meal plan. This recipe provides a filling meal option for women over 40 because it is brimming with protein, fiber, and important nutrients. Quinoa, lean ground turkey, and vibrant bell peppers combine to create a delicious dish with a satisfying combination of flavors and textures. Enjoy the advantages of this hearty dish while promoting your fertility and general health. Good appetite!

Dinner: Grilled Tofu with Stir-Fried Vegetables and Brown Rice

Enjoy the flavorful and nutritious Grilled Tofu with Stir-Fried Vegetables and Brown Rice—a dish that honors the goodness of plant-based ingredients. Tofu that has been grilled, colorful stir-fried vegetables, and nutty brown rice are combined in this dish to make a filling and well-rounded meal. This recipe stuffed with protein, fiber, vitamins, and minerals is a great addition to a fertility diet for women over 40. Let's look at this wholesome plant-powered treat's ingredients, preparation advice, and amazing advantages.

Ingredients:

- Two tablespoons soy sauce (or tamari for a gluten-free option)
- One block of firm tofu.
- Two tablespoons of divided sesame oil
- One teaspoon of minced garlic
- One teaspoon of ginger that has been finely grated
- One tablespoon rice vinegar - 1 tablespoon honey (or maple syrup for a vegan alternative)
- Two cups mixed stir-fried vegetables (such as bell peppers, broccoli, carrots, and snap peas)
- Green onions and sesame seeds as a garnish (optional)

Preparation:

1. Tofu should first be pressed to remove excess moisture during preparation. Place the block of tofu on a fresh kitchen towel or some paper towels. Put a heavy object on top, like a plate, and gently press down. Give it about 20 minutes to sit.

2. Make the marinade while the tofu is being pressed. Combine the soy sauce, one tablespoon of sesame oil, rice vinegar, honey, grated ginger, and garlic in a small bowl. Up until a smooth blend, whisk.

3. Slice or chop the tofu into cubes after pressing it, as you prefer.

4. Pour the marinade over the tofu in a shallow dish, making sure to coat every piece. Let it marinate for at least 15 minutes if you have the time.

5. Turn the heat to medium-high and preheat your grill or pan. To prevent sticking, lightly oil the grill grates.

6. Grill the tofu for 3 to 4 minutes on each side or until it is thoroughly heated and nicely charred. Take it off the grill, then place it aside.

7. Heat the final tablespoon of sesame oil over medium-high heat in a different pan or wok.

8. Add the vegetables for the stir-fry to the pan and cook, stirring frequently, for 3–4 minutes or until they are tender-crisp.

9. Stir-fry the brown rice cooked for two more minutes to bring the flavors together and heat it through.

10. Turn off the heat and serve the grilled tofu with brown rice and stir-fried vegetables.

11. Garnish with sesame seeds and green onions for visual appeal and additional flavor.

Preparation tips:

- You can boost the marinade's flavor by adding a dash of lime juice or a sprinkle of red pepper flakes.

- Use a nonstick grill pan if you don't have access to an outdoor grill.

- Feel free to try various vegetables based on your preferences and what's in season.

- Quinoa or whole wheat couscous can be used instead of brown rice if you prefer a different grain.

- Add extra garnishes to your dish, like chopped cilantro, diced avocado, or a drizzle of sriracha sauce.

Note:

This delicious and nourishing dish, which combines grilled tofu with stir-fried vegetables and brown rice, honors the tastes and advantages of plant-based ingredients. This dish offers crucial nutrients to support fertility and general well-being with its combination of protein-rich tofu, colorful stir-fried vegetables, and wholesome brown rice. Enjoy the delicious plant-powered treat and the advantages of a healthy meal. Good appetite!

Snack: Edamame Beans

If you're looking for a filling and healthy snack, edamame beans are a fantastic choice for older women. They make for a filling snack that is also healthy. Delicious for your health, these young soybeans. When you require a quick energy boost around noon or a high-protein snack to keep you active, edamame beans can be a good choice. The advantages of this nutritious treat, how to make it, and a few pointers should be covered.

Ingredients:

- One cup edamame beans (fresh or frozen)
- Water
- Salt (optional)
- Seasonings (optional): Garlic powder, chili flakes, soy sauce, etc.

Procedure:

1. The first step is to purchase new or frozen edamame beans from your neighborhood grocery store. Obey the directions on the bundle to properly defrost frozen edamame beans.

2. Add salt to a pot of simmering water.

3. Add the edamame beans to the simmering water, cover, and cook for about 5 minutes or until tender. Release the beans, then wash them in cool water to cool them.

4. After the edamame beans have cooled, clean them with a fresh dishtowel or paper towel.

5. Adding delicate salt or other flavors like soy sauce, garlic powder, or stew powder can alter the type of edamame beans you get. Gently toss them so they are completely covered.

How to Eat:

1. The edamame beans must be completely cool before eating them out of a bowl.

2. Hold the pod between your fingers and put the beans in your mouth to eat edamame. Discard the pods.

3. If you're looking for a twist, edamame beans are great on their own or as a protein-rich topping for salads, stir-fries, or grain bowls.

Meal Preparation Tips:

- When adding flavor, take into account a variety of flavors and edamame bean types.

- Prepare many cooked edamame beans and keep them in the refrigerator for an easy-to-grab snack.

- Add edamame beans into dishes of mixed greens, soups, and sautés for added nutritional value.

- Edamame beans are nutritious when Combined with raw vegetables, whole-grain crackers, or nuts.

Note:

Edamame beans are a flexible, satisfying dietary supplement thick bite that has several health benefits. Whether you eat the beans whole or save them for dinner by storing them in the fridge, they will help you meet your daily requirements for essential nutrients and plant-based protein. They aid in maintaining a regular, altered diet as well. Take advantage of the earthy flavor of edamame beans in this nutritious snack to help you reach your fertility and general health objectives. Make wise food selections, learn, and eat well.

Day 7:

Breakfast: Banana Pancakes with Maple Syrup and Walnuts

Start your day with one of these delicious Banana Pancakes with Maple Syrup and Walnuts. This recipe contains the standard pleasantness of bananas with the pound of walnuts and the fertility of maple syrup, making them a healthy and liberal breakfast choice. This recipe gives exemplary pancakes a great makeover while giving more established ladies essential nutrients. These pancakes become a staple in your fertility supper plan thanks to their nutritious fixings and delectable enhancements. Let's start by discussing the dish, some ideas for decorating, and the fantastic advantages of today's early charm.

Ingredients:

- One cup of unsweetened almond milk
- One tablespoon of maple syrup

- One teaspoon of vanilla extract
- One-quarter cup chopped walnuts, coconut oil, or cooking spray for greasing
- One cup whole wheat flour
- One tablespoon of baking powder
- Half teaspoon of ground cinnamon,
- One quarter teaspoon salt.

Procedure:

1. Mix the whole wheat flour, salt, baking soda, cinnamon powder, and mashed banana in a bowl. Stir thoroughly to combine.

2. Combine the almond milk, maple syrup, and vanilla extract in a different bowl.

3. Combine the dry ingredients with the wet ingredients just enough to combine. Remember that a couple of lumps are OK; don't overmix.

4. The chopped walnuts should be gently folded, with a small portion reserved for garnishing.

5. Heat a nonstick griddle or skillet to medium heat. Lightly oil the surface with coconut oil or cooking spray.

6. Using a 1/4 cup measuring cup, scoop the hotcake batter into the skillet and spread it out slightly to form a circle.

7. On each side, cook the pancakes for two to three minutes or until golden brown. With a spatula, flip them tenderly.

8. Remove the pancakes from the skillet and organize them in a stack on a plate.

9. Add more maple syrup to the pancakes and top them with the excess reserved walnuts.

10. At the point when the banana pancakes with maple syrup and walnuts are warm, appreciate their delectable flavors.

Meal Preparation Tips:

- You can upgrade the flavor of the hotcake player by adding a tablespoon of honey or a hint of gritty-shaded sugar.

- Use a variety of garnishes, such as fresh berries, banana slices, or a dollop of Greek yogurt, to add more flavor and surface.

- Incorporate a scoop of your preferred protein powder into the pancakes to boost their protein content.

- Whole wheat flour can be substituted for a gluten-free mixture if you prefer a gluten-free version.

- For future quick and easy morning meals, make a double batch of pancakes and store the extras in the freezer.

Note:

A delicious and filling breakfast option, banana pancakes with maple syrup and walnuts are a sweet addition to your fertility diet. These pancakes are a satisfying way to start the day, thanks to the natural goodness of bananas, the crunch of walnuts, and the fertility of maple syrup. Partake in each nibble, relishing the flavors and supplements. Get ready to eat!

Lunch: Greek Salad with Grilled Chicken and Whole Wheat Pita

Whole-wheat pita bread, crunchy fresh vegetables, and the tenderness of grilled chicken are all part of this dish. This recipe offers a delectable turn on the exemplary Greek plate of mixed greens while giving more seasoned ladies Over 40 admittance to fundamental nutrients. This salad is an excellent addition to your fertility diet due to its healthy ingredients and Mediterranean-inspired flavors. Let's look at the recipe, some tips for making it, and all the great benefits of this filling meal.

Ingredients:

- Two skinless, boneless bosoms of chicken
- Olive oil, one tablespoon
- One teaspoon of dried oregano
- Three tablespoons of extra virgin olive oil
- One tablespoon of red wine vinegar
- One teaspoon of Dijon mustard
- One clove of minced garlic
- Salt and pepper to taste.

- Four cups of mixed salad greens,
- One cup of cherry tomatoes halved
- Half sliced cucumber
- One-quarter of a red onion cut delicately
- One quarter cup Kalamata olives
- One-quarter of a cup of crumbled feta cheese
- Two whole wheat pitas, cut into wedges

Procedure:

1. The temperature of the grill or grill pan should be set to medium-high.

2. Combine the salt, pepper, and dried oregano in a small bowl. Please ensure the chicken breasts are evenly coated by rubbing this mixture over them.

3. The chicken breasts should be grilled on each side for 6 to 8 minutes until they are cooked and no longer pink in the middle. Before being cut into strips, they should be removed from the grill and rest for some time.

4. Mix the mixed salad greens, cucumber slices, red onion, Kalamata olives, and crumbled feta cheese in a large bowl.

5. In a separate small bowl, combine the extra virgin olive oil, red wine vinegar, Dijon mustard, minced garlic, dried oregano, salt, and pepper to make the Greek plate of mixed greens dressing.

6. To uniformly cover the fixings, delicately prepare the plate of mixed greens with the dressing.

7. Place the Grilld chicken fingers on the mixed greens between the plates.

8. Along with the Greek plate of mixed greens and Grilld chicken, serve the whole wheat pita wedges.

Meal Preparation Tips:

- To enhance flavor, marinate the chicken breasts for 30–60–90 minutes to an hour in the olive oil and herb mixture before grilling.

- If you don't have a grill, warm the chicken in the oven or a grill skillet until it is cooked through.

- Add extra ingredients to your salad to make it your own, like artichoke hearts, roasted red pepper slices, or avocado slices.

- To add more crunch, toast the wheat pita wedges on the stove until firm.

Note:

Greek Salad with Grilled Chicken and Whole Wheat Pita is a filling and healthy recipe that uses healthy ingredients and fresh flavors from the Mediterranean. Because of its abundance of fresh vegetables, grilled chicken, and nutritious whole wheat pita bread, this salad provides women over 40 with essential nutrients. Take advantage of the health benefits and indulge in a taste of Greece while enjoying the fusion of flavors. Good luck!

Dinner: Baked Salmon with Lemon-Dill Sauce, Quinoa, and Steamed Asparagus

This recipe is a brilliant and healthy dish for ladies Over 40 since it contains highly nutritious salmon with fresh lemon-dill sauce, the dietary benefit of quinoa, and the delicacy of steamed asparagus. This recipe's flavors and essential nutrients are ideal for women over 40. This meal is a great addition to your fertility meal plan because it contains omega-3 fatty acids, protein, fiber, and vitamins. How about we inspect this scrumptious dish's fixings, fertility directions, and benefits?

Ingredients:
- Two salmon filets
- One meagerly cut lemon
- One tablespoon of additional virgin olive oil
- Salt and pepper to taste
- Fresh dill sprigs as garnish.

For the Dill-Citrus Sauce:

- One cup of quinoa
- Two cups of water or vegetable broth
- Salt to taste for steamed asparagus
- One tablespoon of finely chopped fresh dill
- One-quarter cup of plain Greek yogurt
- Salt and pepper to taste

For the Quinoa:

- One cup quinoa
- Two cups water or vegetable broth
- Salt, to taste

Procedure:

1. Your oven should be preheated to 200°C (400°F).

2. Salmon filets should be placed on a paper baking sheet. Season the salmon with salt and pepper before drizzling it with olive oil.

3. Each salmon fillet should have lemon slices on top. Consequently, the fish will acquire a mild citrus flavor.

4. Bake the salmon for 12 to 15 minutes in a preheated oven or until it flakes easily with a fork.

5. While the salmon heats, set up the lemon-dill sauce by blending Greek yogurt, lemon juice, new dill, minced garlic, salt, and pepper in a little bowl. Combine thoroughly before combining.

6. Bubbling water or vegetable stock should be ready in a pot. Add a touch of salt and the quinoa. Cover and simmer for about 15 minutes, or until the quinoa is fluffy and all the liquid has been absorbed, on low heat. Cover it for an additional five minutes after turning off the intensity.

7. Steam the asparagus in a steamer basket over boiling water. After 5-7 minutes of steaming, the asparagus should be delicate but fresh.

8. Place a portion of cooked quinoa on each plate to begin the meal. Add a salmon filet that has been heated on top. Place the salmon near the steamed asparagus.

9. Embellish the salmon with a couple of new dill branches and a shower of lemon-dill sauce.

10. With lemon wedges on the side, serve the baked salmon with quinoa, steamed asparagus, and a lemon-dill sauce.

Meal Preparation Tips:

- Add spices like dill, parsley, or thyme to give the salmon an additional flavor help before baking.

- Your quinoa dish can contain diced tomatoes, sautéed onions, or bell peppers.

- Assuming you'd prefer to utilize another grain, you can change out the quinoa for brown rice, couscous, or farro.

- Pick firm, new asparagus for steaming. Before using, trim off the tough ends.

Note:

Quinoa and Steamed Asparagus is a nutritious and delicious supper that gives fundamental omega-3 unsaturated fats, protein, fiber, and supplements for ladies Over 40. Savor the savory baked salmon, fluffy quinoa, tender steamed asparagus, and flavorful lemon-dill sauce. This tasty dish won't just satisfy your sense of taste, yet it will likewise support your body. Take advantage of the health benefits and savor every bite. Favorable luck!

Snack: Mixed Fruit Salad with Greek Yogurt

A mixed fruit salad with Greek yogurt is a light and healthy dish that combines a variety of fresh fruits with creamy Greek yogurt. It is a delicious way to enjoy the fruit's vibrant and sweet flavors. This colorful and delightful plate of mixed greens is a delight for your taste buds and a wonderful way to incorporate essential nutrients into your meal plan. This regular item salad upholds your general prosperity and success and provides energy since it contains vitamins, minerals, and cell fortifications. Let's look at the ingredients, how to make it, and the amazing benefits of this delicious dish.

Ingredients:

- One cup of blueberries
- One cup of cut strawberries
- One cup of pineapple chunks
- One cup of divided grapes
- One cup of peeled and chopped kiwis

- One cup of diced and peeled mango
- One cup of Greek yogurt
- Two teaspoons of honey and fresh mint leaves

Procedure:

1. Prepare the fruits by washing, dicing, and halving them as needed. Please place them in a large bowl to mix.

2. Combine the Greek yogurt and honey in a small bowl. Combine thoroughly until the honey is evenly distributed throughout the yogurt.

3. Over the arrangement of natural products in the bowl, spread the yogurt-honey blend. Toss the fruit with the yogurt in a gentle manner until it is all covered.

4. Serve the fruit salad in individual or serving bowls.

5. Embellish with new mint leaves for more flavor and newness.

6. Enjoy the reviving flavors of the Greek yogurt-topped blended organic product salad immediately.

Meal Preparation Tips:

- You can alter the fruit selection based on your preferences and what is in season. Fruits like oranges, pomegranate seeds, blackberries, and raspberries can be added or substituted.

- To preserve their texture and flavor, ensure the fruits are firm but ripe.

- For a creamier surface, utilize full-fat Greek yogurt. Then again, assuming you need something lighter, Greek yogurt with almost no fat is another decision.

- Granola or chopped nuts can eventually be added to the natural product salad to add extra crunch and nutrition.

Note:

A delightful and refreshing dish, blended organic product salad with Greek yogurt joins the regular pleasantness of new natural products with the smoothness of Greek yogurt. Due to its abundance of nutrients, minerals, and cell reinforcements, this salad is an excellent and healthy addition to your fertility dinner plan. Enjoy the myriad flavors, the health benefits, and every spoonful. Get ready to eat!

Extra Methods to Enhance Fertility

A. Hydration:

To keep up with your fertility objectives, it's vital to remain hydrated. The production, distribution, and transportation of nutrients and chemicals are just a few of the physical processes in which water plays a significant role. Attempt to drink something like eight glasses of water every day; You might want to consume more when the weather is hotter, or you exercise. Remember that staying hydrated is essential for improving fertility and preserving general health.

B. Techniques for relaxation and Stress Management

Chronic stress can disrupt hormone balance and impair reproductive function, harming fertility. Consider pressure the board rehearses like thoughtfulness, profound breathing activities, yoga, or participating in agreeable extracurricular exercises. Stress levels can be reduced, and a more balanced and fertile state can be encouraged by creating a calm environment and scheduling time for self-care activities.

C. Regular Physical Activity and Exercise:

Standard active work and exercise meaningfully affect fertility. Exercise improves blood flow, hormone balance, and weight management, lowering the risk of fertility-threatening conditions like polycystic ovary syndrome (PCOS). To establish a long-term routine, choose activities you enjoy and try to get at least 30 minutes of moderate exercise most days of the week.

D. Maintaining a Healthy Body Weight:

Fertility needs to maintain a healthy body weight because excess and underweight can affect chemical levels and the ability to regenerate. Your goal should be a gold BMI within the healthy range (18.5-24.9) and an effort to maintain a reasonable diet that includes food sources high in supplements. To assist you in achieving and maintaining a healthy weight, a specialist in medical services or an employed dietitian can offer you individualized guidance.

Remember that even though these tips can support fertility, you should talk to a fertility-focused doctor or hired dietitian about any specific issues or concerns. You can optimize your fertility journey and increase your chances of conception by implementing a holistic strategy that combines healthy eating, adequate hydration, stress management, regular exercise, and maintaining a healthy weight.

CONCLUSION

Congratulations! You have finished the seven-day fertility meal plan that was made just for women over 40. By combining nutrient-rich food sources, individualized meals, and careful dietary patterns, you have taken significant steps to improve your fertility and overall prosperity. The fundamental targets of this dinner plan were to keep up with weight, balance chemicals, advance regenerative well-being, and give key supplements.

During your fertility journey, you can always try a lot of mouthwatering and filling dishes that use healthy ingredients like leafy greens, lean proteins, whole grains, and bright fruits and vegetables. Sticking to the dinner plan gives your body the fundamental nutrients, minerals, cell reinforcements, omega-3 unsaturated fats, and supplements expected for conceptive well-being and fertility.

Recollect that keeping a healthy, adjusted lifestyle requires continuous exertion. Give reliable activity, supplement-rich food sources, hydration, segment control, and a sound eating routine a first concern to accomplish your fertility objectives. Adopting self-care routines and stress-reduction strategies can improve overall health.

As you push ahead with becoming fertile, contemplate requesting help from clinical experts who know about food and productivity. They can provide you with individualized direction, monitor your progress, and address any particular requirements or concerns you may have.

Be positive, have faith in your body, and believe in the power of food. You can significantly improve your fertility and increase your chances of conception by demonstrating tenacity and perseverance and utilizing the appropriate nutritional support. Kindly leave a positive review about this book and how we can better serve you, as our concern is your health. Thank you for reading, and I hope you share your testimonies nine months from now.

Wishing you the best for your fertility journey, and may the seven-day fertility diet plan lay the groundwork for a prosperous, active, and strong future!

Made in the USA
Las Vegas, NV
16 January 2025